WAKING UP DRY

How to End
Bedwetting Forever

Martin B. Scharf, Ph.D.

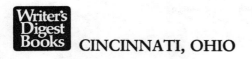 CINCINNATI, OHIO

Library of Congress Cataloging-in-Publication Data

Scharf, Martin, 1946-
  Waking up dry.

  Includes index.
  2. Enuresis—Treatment. I. Title.
RJ476.E6S33 1986   618.92'849   86-19029
ISBN 0-89879-229-0

Design by Sheila Lynch

Dedicated to the memory of my father,
who had the highest hopes for his bedwetter

Acknowledgments

This book could not have been written without the encouragement and support of my wife, Lauren, and children, Rosalyn and Cyvia. The late nights and strange phone calls from very young voices were accepted with patience and understanding.

While many of the techniques used in the bedwetting program came from the work of other researchers and clinicians, the ultimate usage is the result of enormous feedback from parents and the children themselves. Something new continues to be learned from each child, and to them I am truly grateful.

Pat Beusterien spent many hours listening to my taped notes and had to convert them to readable English. My concern is that she will now open her own clinic across the street.

Finally, special thanks to the administrations of the Miami Valley Hospital of Dayton, Ohio, and The Mercy Hospital of Hamilton-Fairfield, Ohio, for their continued support.

Contents

works. An exercise to help your child respond to the alarm. The nighttime training routine. A Dry Nights Star Chart your child can be proud of.

When your child is earning stars for almost-dry nights. Making some modifications in the program. Watch for deconditioning.

When your child is earning stars for dry nights. Phasing out the treatment program. Visual sequencing— a mental rehearsal to help your child stay dry. How to wean your child from the alarm. The relapse possibility.

Consider the causes of the bedwetting. Doing the exercises to stop bedwetting. Restricting caffeinated, carbonated and alcoholic beverages. Importance of using the wetness alarm regularly. Use of the stream-interruption exercises by elderly to help regain bladder control.

Introduction

Waking Up Dry

Several years ago, when very few physicians were paying much attention to bedwetting in terms of treatment, a young lady with a bedwetting problem came to see me. She was eighteen years old and had wet almost every night of her life. She had sought help from specialists and clinics without success. Her parents felt sorry for her and they thought she would probably have the problem for the rest of her life. She was about to go away to college and was frantic because she wanted to live in the dormitory. She thought her bedwetting problem was due to a sleep disorder (which we know now is not the cause in most cases), so she came to me—a sleep disorders specialist—and I agreed to help her.

I began to work with her using some of the current behavior modification techniques, but my concept was to build on existing approaches, rather than simply to follow one approach or another. I wanted to use what I had learned about sleep physiology from research done in our sleep laboratory and in others over a ten-year period.

Despite the fact that at eighteen she was still wetting the bed, this young lady was a very poised, mature, well-adjusted person—the kind of young lady that every parent would love to have as a daughter. She was very cooperative, she was conscientious about carrying out all the steps I suggested, and she responded beautifully to the treatment. It went like clockwork, and she very quickly improved to the point that she has never wet again.

You'd have thought from her reaction that I'd accomplished something that no one else could have done, but in fact, she did it herself.

After this young woman had conquered her condition, I started developing and testing different methods for treating bedwetting and began accepting other people into a bedwetting treatment program.

Eventually, because of the number of people who wanted to enter the program as a result of word-of-mouth recommendations and widespread media coverage, it was necessary to set up a more structured program, so a Bedwetting Clinic became part of the Sleep Disorders Center in Cincinnati.

The people who came to the clinic were very skeptical. They had not responded to other treatments. They had tried everything else, and nothing had worked. Many had even tried some of the things I suggested, such as stream interruption exercises to strengthen bladder muscles, but in a sort of haphazard way, once or twice a day, forgetting that to strengthen any muscle, exercises have to be done in sets and repetitions.

I was amazed at the number of those who responded who had not succeeded elsewhere. The treatment approach, I think, is really quite simple and logical; it just requires patience, and a dose of understanding and reassurance.

Why I Wrote This Book

Bedwetting affects an enormous number of children (and adults, as well), and I'd like to dispel some of the myths concerning it. Unlike what you might read or hear in the media, or be told by those using scare tactics to sell services or products, bedwetting is usually due to merely a maturational lag. However, while most children will outgrow bedwetting (the spontaneous cure rate is 15 percent per year), I think it is unfair to wait for this to happen when the wetting becomes a problem for the child. He must live with shame, embarrassment, teasing by siblings and friends, low self-esteem, and often an unpleasant, even abusive, parent-child relationship. Delaying treatment can be harmful to a child's emotional development; it may present social problems as well (no summer camp, sleepovers, or long trips, for example). For parents, the bedwetting problem can cause guilt, worry, and frustration.

So many parents who bring their children to our Bedwetting Clinic say to me, "I wish there had been a place when I was growing up where I could have gotten treatment," or "I don't want my child to suffer like I did." I know what they mean. As a former bedwetter myself, I personally want to see to it that a lot of children today don't have to grow up with the painful experiences I had.

This book is part of that effort. The treatment described is designed to help the majority of bedwetters. But I also speak of less common types of bedwetting so that you can evaluate what kind of problem you probably face. In particular, it is important to note that bedwetting can be a symptom of a medical condition such as diabetes or a urinary tract infection, and no treatment should be started without first consulting a family physician, pediatrician, or other medical specialist.

Emotional as well as physical causes of bedwetting must also be considered, and psychological assessment of the problem is sometimes indicated.

This book will enable you to understand the bedwetting problem, its causes and effects. It will show you how to treat the problem at home. It is something that can be done at home, and the reason I know this is that I, personally, have treated many children through long-distance telephone calls, serving as a coach.

The treatment program is designed for maximum participation on the part of the child, depending on his or her age. The success of the program depends to a great extent on having the child take as much responsibility for the treatment as possible. Similarly, the older child or the adult can read this book and take full charge of his own treatment.

The treatment program doesn't use aversive, painful kinds of reinforcement. Instead, it focuses on the positive. I would like to see an experience that has been painful turn into something positive, enabling a child to say, "Look what I was able to beat. Look what I was able to overcome, and I worked hard for this."

Bear in mind that in most cases the bedwetting problem is not life-threatening (except if flooding is taking place and the child can't swim), and also that Mother Nature will eventually correct the situation, generally within the lifetime of the parents. This program is designed to speed Mother Nature along.

Style Note: We have used the form "he" and "him" rather than "he/ she" and "him/her" for simplicity and ease of reading, but all references in the book apply to feminine as well as masculine gender.

1

The Nature of the Problem

Bedwetting, or enuresis, is a common childhood (and adult) problem. Estimates are that five to seven million children in the United States wet their beds with regularity, and boys are 50 percent more likely than girls to be affected. A number of studies carried out in our country, Great Britain, Israel, and African countries have demonstrated that approximately 10 percent of all six-year-old children continue to wet their beds and that the spontaneous cure rate thereafter is approximately 15 percent per year. This essentially means that a child who is wetting at age six has a 70 percent chance of continuing to wet at age eight—not the best news for mothers, who are usually the ones involved in changing and washing the sheets, pillow cases, and blankets.

Other statistics show that as many as 1 percent to 3 percent of eighteen-year-olds wet their beds. (In fact, studies of American and British naval recruits have revealed that bedwetting is the number-one cause of rejection from military service.)

All this suggests that bedwetting is an enormous problem, and while not life-threatening, it deserves at least as much attention as the "heartbreak of psoriasis." In fact, although most children outgrow the condition, there can be psychological and social consequences for both the child and the family.

Primary and Secondary Bedwetting

Bedwetting is usually divided into two main categories, primary and secondary. Children with primary bedwetting have never experienced an extended period of dryness (two or three months) without the use of some treatment, such as medication. Bedwetting is secondary in nature when the child has stopped for an extended period of time and subsequently resumes wetting. Statistics show that approximately 90 percent of bedwetting is primary in nature and that 5 percent to 10 percent is secondary.

Causes of Primary Bedwetting

Although both medical and psychological factors can contribute to the problem, the most common causes of *primary* bedwetting are a functional bladder capacity that is too small and an irritable bladder.

Functional bladder capacity is the number of ounces one can hold in the bladder before one feels an urgent need to go to the bathroom. It may not reflect the actual size of the bladder.

When a child (or anyone) feels the need to go to the bathroom, it's the result of a wave of contractions in the walls of the bladder pushing down on the fluid in the bladder. When this happens, a muscle at the bottom of the bladder, the inner sphincter muscle, automatically opens and the only thing left holding back the urine is the outer sphincter muscle, which is under voluntary control. (See illustration on page 9.) The ability of the child to withhold urine depends on the intensity of the bladder contraction: the greater the intensity, the greater the pressure against the outer sphincter muscle.

Some children have very strong bladder contractions, so that even a small amount of urine in the bladder can be put under intense pressure, giving a very strong sense of urgency. This is why, as I said, functional bladder capacity doesn't necessarily reflect the size of the bladder.

Children who wet their beds have been shown to have

stronger bladder contractions than children who don't. We don't know why the contractions are so strong, but it's probably in most cases an inherited trait.

Bladder capacity, of course, is significant in that we want a child to hold urination for as long as ten to twelve hours during the night. If bladder capacity (functional or actual) is below normal for the child's age, then the child must awaken a number of times to go to the bathroom or he will wet the bed. Most parents of bedwetters complain that their children are very deep sleepers and cannot be awakened even by intense prodding. It is no wonder, then, that these children are unable to awaken to signals of a full bladder.

Bladder irritability means there is more than the normal amount of action going on in the bladder: it means there are more and stronger contractions. This may result in a sense of fullness long before actual fullness is reached.

All of us experience frequent bladder contractions during the day, resulting in a sensation of a need to urinate. Our response in most cases is to tighten the outer sphincter muscle, the muscle that voluntarily controls the opening and closing of the bladder. This generally results in a withholding of urination, and over a period of time, the sensation of the need to urinate passes, only to recur again at a future time with a stronger bladder contraction and a greater feeling of urgency. These bladder contractions, as well as urine production, are not limited to waking hours. While urine production is diminished somewhat during sleep, it still exists.

Children who wet the bed have more bladder contractions than children who don't wet the bed. When these occur during very deep sleep, along with the muscle relaxation that also occurs during the deeper stages of sleep, a child is less likely to respond to the contractions and it's "Surf City" time.

As for the underlying cause of these difficulties, genetic factors seem to play a role. Seventy percent of children with primary bedwetting have a family history in which at least one parent or an aunt or uncle had a similar problem.

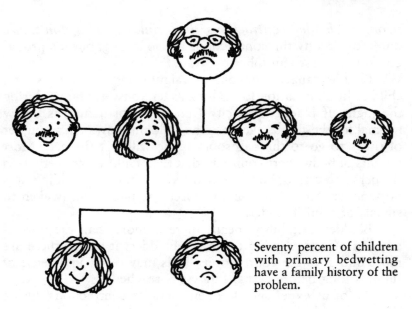

Seventy percent of children
with primary bedwetting
have a family history of the
problem.

HOW THE BLADDER FUNCTIONS

The bladder serves as a storage container for urine (see illustration). It is a triangular-shaped, expandable container. As urine enters, the bladder increases in size; at a certain point, the individual senses pressure and feels the need to urinate. The pressure is felt not only on the walls of the bladder, but also at the lower end of the bladder, where the inner sphincter muscle is located. (We have no control over this muscle.) The pressure of a full bladder leads to the opening of the inner sphincter muscle. Fortunately for us, there is an outer sphincter muscle, which is under *voluntary* control. (If this muscle is weak, it can be strengthened by exercise to withhold larger volumes of urine in the bladder.) Assuming that a certain level of urine is in the bladder, a wave of contraction will occasionally pass through the bladder. This wave of contraction will squeeze the bladder, forcing its contents, the urine, down against the inner sphincter muscle. The inner sphincter muscle then opens, but fortunately

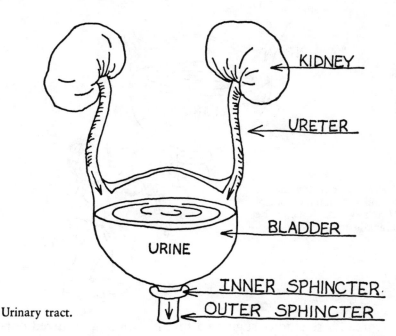

KIDNEY

URETER

BLADDER

URINE

INNER SPHINCTER.

OUTER SPHINCTER

Urinary tract.

we can hold back the urine with the outer sphincter muscle until that wave of contraction completely passes. Once this passes, if we have not opened our outer sphincter muscle— hooray!—we're still dry.

The child with a bedwetting problem does not react to the wave of contraction while asleep. Three methods are used to improve this situation. One is to increase the size of the bladder, thereby lowering the residual level so that the bladder can hold more; another is to increase the awareness of the signals from the wave of bladder contraction. A third method is to increase the tone of the outer sphincter muscle. All three of these methods are used in the treatment program outlined in this book.

BEDWETTING IS NOT A SLEEP DISORDER

Early research on bedwetting suggested that primary bedwet- ting was a disorder of arousal, similar to sleepwalking and night

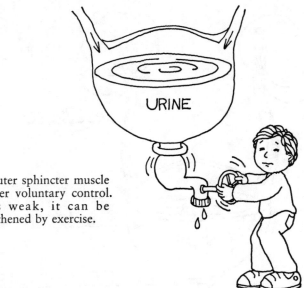

The outer sphincter muscle
is under voluntary control.
If it's weak, it can be
strengthened by exercise.

terrors. These studies suggested that bedwetting occurred during a very deep sleep and was associated with an immature nervous system and specific brain wave patterns reflective of deep sleep. However, subsequent studies carried out in our Sleep Disorders Center, as well as others, have demonstrated that bedwetting can occur in all stages of sleep. Further, it is not related to pathologic deep sleep, nor is it, in fact, a disorder of arousal in the sense of night terrors, nightmares, and sleepwalking. The current thinking is that bedwetting does not ordinarily reflect an abnormality of any sleep stage.

However, knowledge of sleep stages is important in understanding bedwetting.

SLEEP STAGES

Sleep is divided into a series of cycles (see illustration) that all of us pass through during the night. After the first year of life, each cycle tends to last between seventy-five and ninety minutes.

Sleep depth waxes and wanes, and we pass through these cycles as if riding a roller coaster, descending into the deeper stages of sleep and then coming up to a light sleep. Though the sleep patterns of individuals differ, the general pattern is to descend through stages 1, 2, 3, and 4, stage 4 being the deepest, during the first hour of sleep, then to come back up through stages 3 and 2 to the REM (rapid-eye-movement) stage. Both stage 1 and REM sleep are the lightest stages of sleep, but it is in the REM stage that dreaming occurs. As the night progresses, the deeper stages of sleep, 3 and 4, tend to disappear, and a greater proportion of each ninety-minute cycle is spent in the lighter, dreaming (REM) sleep as morning approaches. Conversely, early in the night, a greater proportion of the cycle is spent in stages 3 and 4, that is, in deep sleep.

Sleep Patterns in Childhood

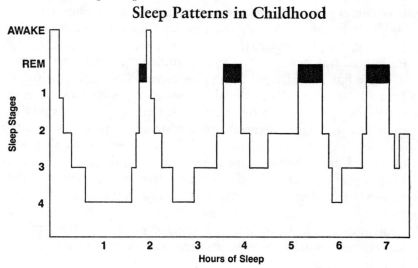

We use this knowledge of sleep cycles to help us treat the bedwetting problem. Part of our strategy is to attempt to shift bedwetting to a later part of the night when sleep is lighter and the child has a greater chance of responding to signals from the bladder. Since most children who wet the bed do so not once

but several times during the night, initial success in treating the
bedwetting problem is in eliminating the later wetting episodes.

SLEEP APNEA—DOES YOUR CHILD SNORE?

An often overlooked factor in the cause of bedwetting is sleep
apnea. Many people, especially those of us who are older, experience pauses in respiration, or episodes of *apnea*. (The term
means absence of breathing.) For most, apnea is related to snoring. When we fall asleep, tissue in our airways relaxes and in
some people vibrates, causing the sound of snoring. Loud snoring suggests the presence of more loose tissue. In certain situations, the airway becomes blocked, causing episodes called *obstructive sleep apnea*. One way to find out if obstructive apnea
is occurring is to listen to snoring. Listen for a pause that is
suddenly followed by a snorting noise. Whenever you hear that
snorting, gasping noise, it is a pretty good indication that the
individual has not been breathing immediately prior to that.

We have considered this a phenomenon occurring primarily in adults, especially older adults, for as tissue loosens, snoring
increases. But now a generation of children is growing up with
their tonsils intact. Whereas we used to often take out tonsils,
now it's rare to do so. Many children have tonsils that are
oversized, that are blocking the airway, and these children are
loud snorers. Parents should recognize that this is disrupting the
continuity of sleep. We find that these children are very difficult
to awaken in the morning; also, they are often not in a very
good mood. They complain of being tired during the day, or
sometimes actually become hyperactive in a paradoxical response to their fatigue.

In many instances, removing tonsils has cured a child's
bedwetting. If the continuity of a child's sleep is being disturbed
by snoring, when the child does sleep, the sleep is so deep that
he cannot respond to signals from a full bladder. Also, the child
experiencing apnea is not getting adequate oxygen. And oxygen
loss and the decrease in oxygen levels, what we call *desatura-*

tion, then decrease the responsiveness of that child, and depending how severe it is, may lead to episodes of bedwetting. I have worked with a number of children who were found to have apnea, and after they were treated, the bedwetting was resolved as well.

So, although apnea is not usually a major factor in bedwetting, it is certainly something that needs to be looked at. It is logical to focus on the bladder and the urologic systems when looking for causes of bedwetting, but strange as it may seem, a problem with bedwetting can originate in the throat. In fact, anything that disrupts sleep may contribute to bedwetting.

If you suspect that your child may have apnea, you need to discuss the problem with a physician and consider a consultation with a sleep-disorders specialist.

FOOD ALLERGY AND BEDWETTING

Another factor that may contribute to bedwetting is food allergy. It is suggested that some children with allergy to milk will improve in their bedwetting problem as soon as afternoon and evening milk is eliminated from their diet. We do not completely understand this, but I have seen this result in a number of children who have a history of milk allergy.

Causes of Secondary Bedwetting

While most bedwetting is primary in nature—children have never experienced an extended period of dryness without some treatment—factors such as diabetes, urinary tract abnormalities, anatomic abnormalities, and psychological factors can result in *secondary bedwetting*, in which previously dry children begin to wet again. Fortunately, only five to ten percent of bedwetting is secondary in nature and likely to involve such factors.

In a study in 1981 of parental perceptions of bedwetting, it was found that 36 percent of the parents surveyed thought that bedwetting was caused by emotional problems; they considered bedwetting to be emotional in origin, and emotional factors were attributed as second only to deep sleep as the major contributing factor in bedwetting. While we know that these perceptions are incorrect, some psychological factors can be significant. For example, when another baby comes into the family and the older child wants attention, he may begin bedwetting. Even though the attention he gets from bedwetting may be negative, it is still attention.

Sometimes anger can cause a child to wet. Sometimes a child will use bedwetting to avoid certain situations such as sleeping over at someone else's house.

Many times a clue that psychological factors are playing a significant role in bedwetting is that a child who has no structural abnormalities in the urinary tract and who did not previously wet begins wetting in the daytime as well as at night.

Effects of Bedwetting

There are very clear social limitations on children who wet their beds. I think of how many parents sneak out of motel rooms leaving evidence of their little visit behind. It is difficult not to share their frustration and their concern with their child. How unfair!

There are social problems in terms of whether a child can sleep away from home and where the child can visit. There has to be a confession of the child's problem and a negotiation before the child can agree to stay over at a friend's or relative's house. This can be so humiliating that it is usually very important to start treatment once this kind of social interaction is likely to occur.

There is no question that, from a psychological standpoint, there are feelings of guilt and shame associated with bedwetting, as well as a feeling of failure of not having reached an appropriate level of maturity. It is very hard for children to appreciate the fact that they have no control over this whatsoever. This is

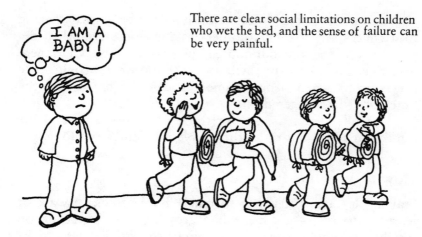

There are clear social limitations on children who wet the bed, and the sense of failure can be very painful.

especially true for a seven- or eight-year-old who has younger brothers or sisters who don't wet the bed. You can tell them that it is not their fault and they may accept it, but every time they fail, it is exactly that—a failure.

Sometimes the sense of failure can be terribly painful. In many instances, parents require children to continue wearing diapers at bedtime until dryness is achieved, thereby constantly reminding the children of their shortcomings. Siblings and friends are often cruel in making fun of the bedwetting child.

In my own situation, there are quite a few memories that have lingered for these thirty or so years since I stopped wetting, despite the fact that my parents were generally kind regarding my problem. Clearly, a less understanding reaction may do considerable damage.

One of the difficulties, however, in trying always to be understanding is that bedwetting puts pressure on the whole family. When the mother has to wake up each morning to face a load of laundry consisting of sheets, blankets, pillow cases, and wet pajamas, it puts a damper on the day. The problem can also be a source of sibling conflict. Even my own father used to tease me about my bedwetting and would often tell me that I was going to wet until I got married. I found myself looking for a wife as a ten-year-old child! Seriously, it can be quite damaging to a child's self-esteem. Another situation occurred when my parents were showing our house to prospective buyers and there was a need to air out my bedroom each morning. I could sense the concern when people came through the house and the "memory" had lingered on.

For all these reasons—for the sake of the child and the family—it's best not to let the problem continue too long.

How to View the Problem

Staying dry at night is not so much like learning to walk or learning to read—it's more like growing tall or putting on weight. In other words, overcoming bedwetting ought to be looked at as a maturational kind of thing at least until the child is about age six. There are certain kinds of things that probably won't surprise you. If one or both parents were bedwetters, don't be surprised if your child is still wetting at age four or five. You certainly wouldn't be surprised if blue-eyed parents had a child with blue eyes.

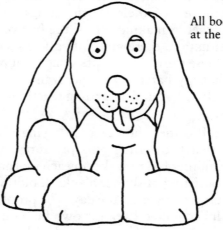

All body parts don't grow at the same rate.

Staying dry all night is the kind of thing a person grows into, not the kind of thing that you can control by adjusting the environment. Not all children mature at the same rate, nor do all body parts grow at the same rate. I ask kids if they have a dog at home and if they've ever seen a puppy dog with really big ears and really big feet. One of the things that you know about that dog is that its feet are too big: its paws have grown faster than the rest of its body. Well, sometimes in a child's body, the ability to produce urine grows faster than the size of the bladder to hold it. Sometimes it takes just a little growth of the bladder to catch up.

Be assured that your child is not wetting the bed on purpose. You need to appreciate that it isn't something intentional and that eventually the problem will be resolved.

Parents become frustrated because they have to change wet sheets and blankets and do extra laundry. They are frustrated over the failure of their child to get dry. Part of that is feeling sorry for the child. But sometimes they feel the child doesn't care, that he isn't complying with the things they think will get him dry: going to the bathroom before bedtime and restricting fluids in the evening (although very rarely does restricting fluids make any difference).

Parents need to have patience and understanding, to appreciate that primary bedwetting is usually due to a maturational lag. They would not be so frustrated or angry if the child had a problem with walking or speech that the doctor said he would outgrow.

It's important to discuss with your child what causes bedwetting, but unless treatment is about to begin, you really need to refrain from pressuring your child to stay dry when this is really a physical impossibility. And you should realize that training should not be started until the child is old enough to want to stay dry and to take an active part in and responsibility for the treatment, and that is usually around age six.

Q. Is bedwetting a modern problem?

A. No, bedwetting has persisted from time immemorial. In fact, one of the earliest known writings about it was in 1550 B.C. *Papyrus Ebers*, an ancient Egyptian medical text, described the use of Juniper berries, cypress, and beer as a treatment for curing bedwetting. (Very few of our kids are guzzling beer to cure this bedwetting today. Most adults, however, would concede that beer can make you aware of signals from a full bladder.) Three thousand years later, the treatments were even more bizarre, for example, a powder prepared from the testicles of a hedgehog or the claws of a goat. In primitive societies, children who wet have sometimes received harsh treatment. Their backsides were blistered, penile ligatures were applied, hot liquids were poured on them.

This is a problem that occurs throughout the world and has occurred throughout time—probably parents of cave children were just as disturbed about it. When their child wet on the bearskin, they didn't have drycleaning to get rid of that smell, and bearskins weren't that easy to get. And they couldn't just find a new cave. So, when today's Moms and Dads begin to feel the pressure of the bedwetting problem, they have to put it in perspective. We have dealt with this problem forever.

Q. Would you describe a typical treatment for sleep apnea in children?

A. I recently worked with an eight-year-old child in our Sleep Disorders Center. He had a rather guttural sound to his breathing, and his mother disclosed that he snored loudly each night and that his snoring was punctuated by gasping and snorting noises. He was also extremely difficult to awaken in the morning. I suggested that he might have sleep apnea and that monitoring in a sleep laboratory would reveal the number and severity of the apneic episodes. She discussed the results of the lab report with her pediatrician, and was then referred to a local children's hospital for further evaluation.

The pediatric otolaryngologist at the hospital found that the child's tonsils were of normal size, and felt strongly that the adenoids were probably similarly normal. But subsequent X-ray revealed the adenoids to be the size of golf balls; they were removed. Within approximately three weeks, the child was staying dry more than 50 percent of the time, and with further work, he was completely and rapidly cured of his bedwetting.

I estimate that as many as five percent of the children who wet the bed have a history of snoring, which should be evaluated by a medical or sleep-disorders specialist.

Q. Is bedwetting sometimes the result of a dream?

A. Children often report bedwetting episodes in which they dream of being in the bathroom and subsequently wet the bed. Many sleep investigators now believe that the wetting has already occurred, or is occurring, at the time of the dream, and that the wetness stimulates the dream and is incorporated into it. In other words, the child starts to wet while in dreaming sleep, the wetness triggers a mental image of being in the bathroom, and the child is suddenly aware of the fact that he is wetting inappropriately. While the data are difficult to argue with, as a former bedwetter, I must insist that I had experiences in which I was dreaming that I was in the bathroom and then I wet.

Q. I get very angry, tense, and frustrated with my child when he continues to wet the bed. My child gets frightened and upset. What can I do to stay calm in this situation?

A. Even under the best of circumstances, with the most understanding parents, there are episodes of frustration and anger. In my own family situation, while my mother dealt very kindly, understandingly, and in a low-key fashion with my bedwetting, she at times got quite upset with having to deal with my soaking sheets and odoriferous room.

First, be assured that your child is not wetting the bed on purpose. Second, ask yourself why you are angry, why you are frustrated. Probably you're upset because you have to change the bed and do the laundry. It is certainly appropriate to have your child take some responsibility by helping to do these things, and doing so may defuse your anger.

Q. Why are parents reluctant to talk about the bedwetting problem?

A. Some parents see bedwetting as a parental failure. Others see it as a shortcoming in their children. Many parents who call me find it difficult to accept that their "little gems," who have crawled and walked earlier than any of their friends' children, who have learned to read almost while in utero, and who are unquestionably the future presidents, congressmen, and leaders of this country, can have this major blemish on their climb to the top by failing to overcome bedwetting. How enlightening it would be if we were to discover that Alexander the Great was still a bedwetter when he conquered Asia!

Bedwetting is indeed a private problem within the family and probably shouldn't be discussed freely in front of outsiders. But parents ought at least to be sure that their children understand the problem so that they can deal with it effectively. Some of our teenage bedwetters have a better understanding of why they have pimples than they do of why they wet the bed.

Parents often do not even mention bedwetting to the pediatrician. As a result, most children are not aware that their problem is not unique, and they have little insight into what causes it or when or how it may be overcome.

Q. How sensitive are children about their bedwetting?

A. Let me give you an example. I will never forget wetting a friend's bed as a child. This particular friend had been a bedwetter, and he and I both knew of our mutual problem, but he outgrew it before I did. It was quite rare for me to spend the night at anyone else's house, but I agreed to spend the night at this friend's house.

I remember vividly my concern. At that time, my bedwetting was somewhat sporadic and not occurring every night. I woke up at 2:00 in the morning, and to my horror, with a sinking feeling, found that I had wet his bed. For the rest of the night, I cowered in the corner of the bed with the sheets exposed to the air, hoping that they would dry by morning. By the dawn's early light, it looked like they had dried; I didn't see any sign of urine, and I never told anyone. I felt like I had gotten a reprieve from the embarrassment.

About two days later, I overheard my mother and my friend's mother laughing about the fact that I had wet the bed. I was so mortified. My privacy had been invaded. This incident happened probably thirty or thirty-one years ago, and I still vividly remember it. There was nothing malicious in their conversation. I'm sure they had no idea that I had overheard, and probably had no idea that I was so sensitive, but it was one of the few times that I spent the night away from home, and it was a disaster.

You need to be sensitive to your child and ask whether it is OK to discuss the problem. It is one thing to discuss it with a doctor, but it is another to discuss it with friends, especially in the presence of the child. And it *really* is an embarrassment when you are speaking with the parents of your child's friends. After age five or six, kids are just very, very sensitive. At age four, I think most children are oblivious to the issue unless it is repeatedly pointed out to them.

Most parents who have children who wet the bed were

either bedwetters themselves or have someone in their family who used to wet the bed. Try to remember how painful this problem was for you or for your brother or sister. This helps to evoke some compassion and sensitivity.

Q. Will it help to tell my child about the hereditary factor in bedwetting?

A. Yes, it does help your child to know that this is not some kind of bad habit he has developed by himself. But it isn't enough to tell a child, "Well, your Dad wet until he was twelve." If this is a six-year-old child, he may be thinking about being wet for longer than he's been alive! What I prefer to do is to tell the child, "Your Dad wet until he was twelve. You're six now, and we are going to see to it that you beat your Dad." That always brings a smile to a child's face. All kids like to think that they can surpass their parents in some way.

Q. What are some of the most common reasons children give for wanting to overcome bedwetting? Do these change with the age of the child?

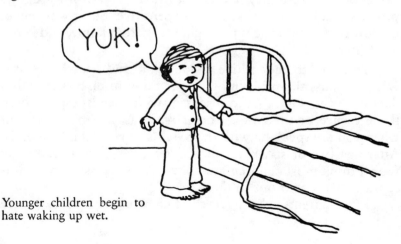

Younger children begin to hate waking up wet.

A. Frankly, what most children say is, "It's yukky!" They begin to hate waking up wet—it smells and it's cold. They can't spend the night at someone else's house because they'd be embarrassed if they wet the bed. They also see bedwetting as a sign of failure on their part. It's very hard to feel grown up when they're still saddled with a behavior of infancy.

Of course, feelings do change with the age of the child. Younger children feel frustration but they really don't see the scope of the problem. Children of eleven or twelve begin to feel that the problem is *never* going to go away, and it greatly contributes to a sense of insecurity. All the problems and insecurities of puberty are magnified when a child is still wetting the bed.

Older children feel that the problem is *never* going to go away.

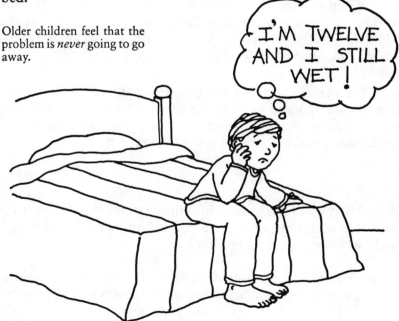

Q. What can I do to keep my child from being embarrassed about his problem?

A. You need to be very sensitive to your child's feelings. For example, if your child is wetting the bed regularly, you need to discuss with him whether or not he wants to have somebody sleep over, or whether or not he wants to sleep at someone else's house. If the family is going to Grandma's house, how does the child feel? If it will be a problem, what can he do? Does he want anyone to know that he has this problem? Try to be very accommodating to the wishes of your child.

Some practical adjustments may make social visits easier, such as taking a special sleeping bag with a rubber sheet in it, or bringing a pad and an extra sheet to protect the bed your child will sleep in. The aim is to maintain privacy and discretion. It is very, very important that your child's feelings be sheltered.

When you are traveling, be prepared for an accident so that it doesn't become a big deal. Pack your own rubber pad and sheet for the motel bed, or make sure that you awaken your child a number of times during the night to take him to the bathroom.

Doing these practical things and keeping the problem in the family—as opposed to having a child wet someone else's bed, which in my own experience was really a devastating experience—are gestures your child will be grateful for.

Q. How can I make my child understand that bedwetting is not a complete disaster to be ashamed of but a simple problem we can fix together?

A. You can talk to your child about the reasons for bedwetting, perhaps the family history of the problem. Explain that some kids get dry faster just as some kids get tall faster. Tell him that there are some things he can do to try to solve the problem, that other kids have the same frustration, and that the problem can be treated. Even though it may take a while, he will be able to see steady improvement, and eventually he will stay dry all night.

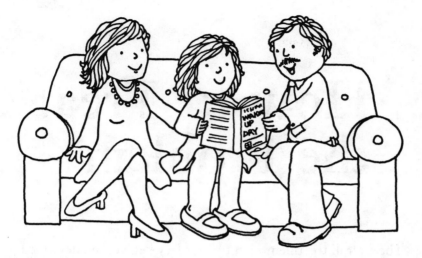

Talk to your child about the reasons for bedwetting and how you can solve the problem together.

2

How to Treat the Problem

The overall treatment plan for primary bedwetting described in this book incorporates a number of treatment methods which have been well established as effective to various degrees. They include *bladder stretching and stream interruption, motivational counseling, conditioning,* and *visual sequencing,* or *rehearsal.* (Most clinicians treating bedwetting will use one or more of these treatment methods, but use each method separately rather than putting them all into effect simultaneously.)

As I've said, the treatment outlined here is not for the kind of bedwetting resulting from underlying medical conditions like diabetes, urinary tract infections, or anatomic abnormalities. It is very important to start any bedwetting treatment with a physical examination and a discussion with the family physician to ascertain that medical factors have been ruled out as causes.

If bedwetting has never stopped, it is not very likely that psychological causes are playing a primary role. If there is a lot of stress at home, if parents are not getting along, or the like, that can complicate the problem. But the most serious indication that psychological help is needed is a recurrence of wetting in a child who previously stopped and who has no medical factors that cause wetting.

When to Treat the Bedwetting Problem

Over the past few years, our Bedwetting Clinic has received international attention. I have received literally hundreds of phone calls from mothers of children who are three, four, or five years old, telling me, "My kid talked at an early age and walked at an early age, and can read, type forty words per minute, and do whatever, but still wets the bed, and I know it is really having an effect on the child."

It is very hard for me to appreciate how a four-year-old child can be impaired by bedwetting. When the child is that young, it is important to recognize that the problem is more yours than your child's and that you really need to cool it.

The concern we have with focusing on bedwetting at an early age is that the issue of being wet or dry gets tied into good or bad: "I'm a good child because I was dry this morning."

There is no question that children look for reinforcement. They'll boast that they did something, but their pride in an accomplishment should have nothing to do with whether they are good or bad. Also, parents should not equate getting dry with getting an "A" in school, learning to read, or anything that results from concentrating and trying; staying dry is something that is going to occur naturally. Parents don't brag, "Well, my child is up to four feet," or "My child is up to thirty pounds." They don't focus so much on their child's physical changes as they do on accomplishments, and staying dry needs to be looked at as just one of the physical changes.

So, while your child is too young to appreciate the problem or do anything about it, you need to relax and give your child a chance to grow out of it. As a clinician I want to make sure that the person I'm treating is the child, not the parents, and I don't want to initiate treatment until the wetting becomes an issue for the child.

You don't treat the problem until it really is a problem— for example, when siblings are teasing the child or he can't sleep at a friend's or go to camp. But these kinds of things tend not to happen until the child is at least close to six years old.

Most children are still wetting at age three. And then between ages three and six, there is a decrease in wetting, down to about 10 percent of the kids by age six. So there is a great deal to be said for letting nature take its course for a year or two.

Another consideration, besides when to treat, is whether or not a child is treatable. I don't know if a child is really treatable at age four. The child's bladder may not be mature enough to be able to respond, and one can do more damage by trying to treat a child who is not ready. Also, not all four-year-olds can do some of the exercises, so you might have to wait until their bodies catch up with their IQs.

On the other hand, although usually I don't like to begin treatment until a child is six, I do consider the parental response and the structure of the family; some parents are just not able to be laid back about bedwetting. They simply cannot ignore it. It bothers the heck out of them. As a result, for their own health and for the quality of their parenting and the quality of their future relationship with their child, something has to be done. Under those conditions, I say go ahead and let's get this kid treated, but you must have the patience to help your child understand what you want him to do.

If there is more than one child in the family wetting the bed, I strongly feel that the older child should be treated first and that two children should not be treated simultaneously. The reasons for this are that the older child may feel that he has failed for a longer period of time, and the results can be quite damaging if the younger child becomes dry before the older. Once the older child has achieved a certain level of success, one can begin bladder-stretching and stream-interruption exercises with the younger child.

An Outline of the Treatment Program

The treatment program is directed toward (1) increasing bladder capacity, (2) increasing awareness of signals from a full bladder, and (3) increasing the ability to respond to a bladder contraction by using the outer sphincter muscle to withhold urine.

We want the child to respond to a bladder contraction despite the fact that he is not awake, to respond on a subliminal level. We want the child who is very, very deeply asleep to respond easily. To do that, the child virtually has to have what I call a *hair-trigger sphincter muscle*. I tell the kids that they have to be able to stop on a dime and leave nine cents change. So, the key elements in the initial treatment, consisting of bladder stretching and stream-interruption exercises, are directed toward that goal. Studies done at Johns Hopkins University have shown that the exercises are an effective treatment for as many as 30 percent of the kids who do them. In other words, 30 percent of all bedwetters are going to get dry just from doing these exercises and nothing else. This is a very promising percentage.

Following is an outline of the steps that will be taken in the treatment program:

- Charting relevant activities, such as the number of the child's daytime trips to the bathroom and the time he goes to bed

- Monitoring the child's evening snacks and foods for items that may be bladder irritants, which increase the possibility of bedwetting

- Bladder-stretching (withholding) exercise (to increase capacity of bladder and awareness of a full bladder)

- Midstream-interruption (push-up, or stop-start) exercise (to strengthen the outer sphincter muscle and increase the ability to hold back urination)

- Measurements of bladder capacity (to determine the initial bladder capacity and to monitor increases in capacity as a result of exercises; the process also increases awareness of signals from a full bladder)

- Use of alarm activated by nighttime wetness (to condition the child to respond to bladder contractions and signals from a full bladder)
- Paired-association exercise (practicing midstream-interruption exercise in response to the wetness alarm)
- Visual sequencing, or rehearsal (a conditioning practice that helps the child respond appropriately to bladder contractions and to signals from a full bladder)

The foregoing steps will be discussed in detail as they are introduced in the Step-by-Step Program. The treatment, which is divided into four phases, takes an average of three months (although if a child is wetting several times a night, it may take considerably longer), but improvements can be noticed even in the early stages of the program.

How to Get Your Child to Cooperate

Any attempt at treatment requires compliance with the treatment, and compliance requires motivation. Motivational counseling must be done by whoever is going to handle the treatment—and it should be someone who is not going to get angry with failure or show frustration.

At the beginning of treatment, I usually ask the child to discuss how much he hates his bedwetting and to talk about the problems that bedwetting causes for him, such as difficulty in sleeping at a friend's house, the embarrassment of having friends find out, the unpleasantness associated with siblings making fun of him, or the anger and frustration that his parents have in dealing with wet sheets, blankets, and pillow cases. Even the most embarrassed children frequently become very animated in discussing such problems when I touch the right nerve.

Most children are motivated by a desire to be dry, but sustaining motivation until they are dry can be difficult and requires tremendous energy. And without motivation, the treatment will probably fail, for the child must do some of the work on his own. You can't supervise every stream-interruption exercise, for example, and that is really where the success begins.

As a counselor, it is important that you have a positive attitude, and you should reassure your child that he can expect success. Look very hard for signs of success in the treatment, and be sure to reward *trying*. If all you do is focus on wet or dry, you may overlook signs of trying. Following are some elements of the treatment program that reflect effort on the part of the child: performance of the stream-interruption exercises; extending the period urine is held in the withholding exercise; reducing the size of the wet spot on the bed, which indicates improvement, movement toward success. There are many small steps that a child may take before actually achieving dryness that show that he is indeed trying, and those steps deserve to be rewarded. And rewarding often provides further motivation.

If treatment is delayed until your child wants to get dry, further motivation shouldn't be too difficult. If your child is not interested at all, maybe he is too young. Even at six or seven, he might be emotionally too young. But look at the larger picture: if your child is doing well in school and there are no behavior problems, he is probably well enough adjusted emotionally and socially to begin treatment and to be motivated to stick with it.

Compliance in the treatment requires that your child have a certain amount of self-discipline; however, you should help him to understand that he should expect a series of little successes rather than a sudden big success. If your child is looking only for a dry bed, and he doesn't get the dry bed in the first few weeks of the program, he may stop trying or lose some of his motivation. You can help him to focus on stages of improvement: the stream-interruption exercise is easier to do, or he has a slight increase in bladder capacity, or the number of trips to the bathroom during the day has decreased, for example. He should be told and believe that these are successes. And success tends to breed success.

So, your child needs to work toward the final goal of staying dry all night, but with the smaller successes recognized and
appreciated.

Rewards to Encourage Your Child

At the beginning of the treatment, you and your child might
agree on what reward he will receive when he gets dry. That
might be something like a special toy, a new bed, or a bedroom
set—something very meaningful. However, you shouldn't con-
fuse your child by discussing numerous and various rewards;
instead, focus on a reward for the next tiny step. For example,
you might tell your child, "If you have an increase in the bladder
capacity measurement, we're going to give you a dollar," or "If
you do your exercises every day, we're going to go out and get
an ice cream cone." This sets up a small reward for a small step.
The rewards should be small, but provide immediate gratifica-
tion, something as simple as a small toy, a candy bar, a dollar
bill. They should be things that your child can see and enjoy
directly without having to share with a brother or sister. Asking
a child to stop and start urinating in midstream (there are many
adults who wouldn't do this for any amount of money), asking
a child to hold urine as long as he can and to bear the discomfort—you have to have something awfully sweet at the end for
the child to bear what can border on pain. You need a reinforcement system, and the reward has to be something that says,
"Gee Whiz! you're doing great! I've got something here for you
because you're making progress."

Of course, you should take every opportunity to praise and
encourage your child, to hug him and tell him how well he's
doing, but I wouldn't recommend that at each point you spend a
long time on reinforcement. You can tell him, "Really nice job!"
or "Great going! Let's see how we do tonight," and then period-
ically offer a little more encouragement by giving a reward.

I recommend moderation here because if you put too much
effort into rewarding your child for successes, the disparity dur-

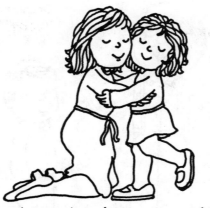

Take every opportunity to praise and encourage your child.

ing times of failure will be too great.

Twenty-five percent of the children with a bedwetting problem respond simply to motivation and reassurance, and if you can properly motivate your child, it will certainly help.

Q. Who else besides parents can help in the treatment?

A. Grandparents can often help with this program in that they have a natural bond with the child. There is a strong element of trust, and the grandparents do not find the bedwetting as frustrating as Mom and Dad do. Another reason grandparents are often ideal implementers of this program is that this is truly a gift of love that the grandparents can provide to their grandchildren, helping them overcome a very difficult problem. Possibly grandparents felt frustrated with their own children's bedwetting, and now they have a second chance—to help make things easier for their grandchildren.

Older siblings, especially a roommate who may be teasing and really putting pressure on the child, can also help. Sometimes I name an offending brother or sister, the one who is really doing the teasing, as the *facilitator*. Like in the *Wizard of Oz*, it

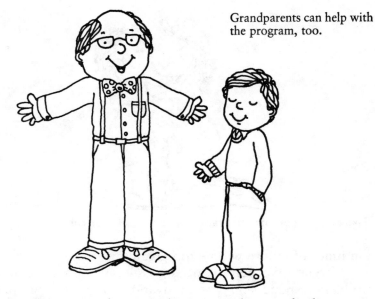

Grandparents can help with the program, too.

is very important to have a title. I name them as facilitators in that they are responsible to see to it that the child does things like the paired-association exercises or the stream-interruption exercises, and they get to share in the rewards when the child is dry. The sibling's involvement actually enhances their relationship in many instances.

But the choice as to whether or not a sibling is to be a facilitator belongs to the child starting treatment. If you decide you are going to reward the older brother or sister, the bedwetting child must clearly understand and agree to the arrangement. I usually get him involved in the decision so that he understands that this is to his benefit as well—big brother or sister is now going to get off his back and in fact is going to turn out to be a helper. So, helping with the treatment can be done by parents, but also by others. In particular, I try to enlist somebody not too emotional about the problem.

Before getting into the details of this treatment for primary bedwetting, however, you may wonder what other treatment methods are available.

Other Treatment Methods:

Medications—How They Work

The number-one treatment that has been used by pediatricians and family physicians is a pharmacologic approach, the use of drugs, and the primary drug prescribed is Tofranil (generic name, Imipramine). Tofranil, an antidepressant, is most frequently used to treat patients with mood disorders, in particular, depression. Most drugs have more than one effect, and the same is true for Tofranil, which also has an anticholinergic effect. This means that it blocks the effects of acetylcholine, a chemical that makes some of the body's nerves function.

In a study that I was involved in some years ago, it was demonstrated that the reason Tofranil can in some cases alleviate bedwetting is that it evidently reduces the irritability of the bladder, possibly through its anticholinergic action. So children on this drug may experience less frequent or less intense bladder contractions during the night

One of the reasons we concluded that Tofranil has a direct effect on the bladder is that we saw some children who were taking standard doses of Tofranil who were not only dry at night but who could not urinate during the day either. Simply lowering the dose (which is given primarily at night) restored their control of daytime urination.

Tofranil is quite effective. In fact, it has an approximately 75 percent success rate in controlling bedwetting. However, it is not a treatment, because only 5 percent to 10 percent of all children who are treated with Tofranil stay dry when the medication is stopped. Instead, there is frequently a rebound: bedwetting actually worsens when the drug is withdrawn for a brief period. So what we have is a finger in the dike, if you will, that works as long as you are standing there against the dam, but as soon as you walk away, you have a gusher on your hands, and that is probably not a bad description. As a result, Tofranil is often recommended for a child who is going to go to camp, who is going to have some friends over, and may be in a very short, transient kind of potentially embarrassing situation in which bedwetting needs to be controlled. But I do not recommend, nor do most clinicians recommend, the use of Tofranil chronically as a treatment for bedwetting in a child.

Another medication that may work in a similar way is called Ditropan. Ditropan and Tofranil are probably the two most frequently used medications for bedwetting.

Behavioral Therapy—Dry-Bed Training

Dry-bed training is the name of a behavioral treatment for bedwetting. It consists of the following four procedures: a nightly waking schedule, positive practice, the use of an alarm set off by wetness, and cleanliness training.

In the nightly waking schedule, the child is awakened every hour until midnight or 1:00 a.m. to go to the bathroom during the first night of training; on subsequent nights, the child is awakened once a night, and the awakening time is adjusted from approximately three hours after bedtime to two-and-a-half, one-and-a-half, and one hour after bedtime, assuming that the child is dry for the remainder of the night. If the child wets twice in one week, the cycle of once-a-night waking starts over, with the child being awakened three hours after he goes to bed.

In the positive practice, the child must lie down on his bed at bedtime and count to fifty, get up and go to the bathroom, and try to urinate. He repeats this procedure approximately twenty times, and does so not only before going to bed, but each time that he experiences a wet bed. The use of a bell and pad that provide an automatic signal when the child starts wetting the bed is not an essential part of this program, but obviously is quite helpful in determining when the child wets and therefore when positive practice should be done.

Cleanliness training is simply having the child be responsible for placing all wet bedding in the laundry hamper and remaking the bed.

Some studies suggest that there are a large number of dropouts from this program because parents find some of the techniques to be quite aversive. However, a fairly large percentage of children eventually get dry with this program. It is a very well established and respected approach to treatment and is certainly something that can be tried. It differs from the approach recommended in this book primarily in that it tends to focus on negative reinforcement rather than positive. For more information about dry-bed training, refer to the book, *A Parent's Guide to Bedwetting Control*, by Nathan H. Azrin, Ph.D., and Victoria A. Besalel, Ph.D.

Hypnosis—An Effective Treatment?

Hypnosis has been reported to be effective in some children. This is not entirely surprising when one understands that hypnosis is a form of meditation, and basically, all hypnosis is really self-hypnosis. If it can increase the child's physical awareness, then that is terrific. I often have children do *visual sequencing*, that is, before going to bed, think quite hard about what they are going to do when they feel the need to go to the bathroom. If they can do this visual sequencing in a very relaxed atmosphere, it sometimes can have the same benefit as is reported for hypnosis.

However, although using hypnosis may help a child respond to a bladder contraction, it will not replace stream-interruption and bladder-stretching exercises. The child must have a strong outer sphincter muscle and the bladder capacity that will enable him to withhold urination through the night.

Urologic Procedures—When Are They Used?

A urologist sometimes finds in a child an abnormal *meatus* (the channel from the urethra to the outside). In particular, the abnormality is a meatal *stenosis* (a narrowing of the opening at the end of the urethra). Many children are born with this condition, and sometimes just by examination one can see that the opening

is too narrow. Such an opening can result in incomplete emptying of the bladder. The surgical treatment for this is called a
meatotomy (cutting and enlarging of the meatus). Sometimes
children undergo cystoscopy, which is the insertion of a cysto-
scope through the urethra to stretch this canal and open any
blockage.

Bedwetting is very occasionally a result of urethral
problems. I see a physical or urologic problem in less than 10
percent of children who wet the bed, and in a smaller percentage
of those cases, I see situations where a urologic procedure is
helpful in eliminating bedwetting.

Psychotherapy—When Is It Necessary?

Children who wet their beds are sometimes referred to psycho-
therapists. However, most psychotherapy lasts for periods of
months or years, and bedwetting is usually self-limiting. We can
expect that a child will almost always outgrow bedwetting over
a period of years. If a child is well adjusted and doing well in
other areas, no psychological evaluation is indicated. But sometimes a child who is being treated for primary bedwetting may
have other problems as well, and psychotherapy may be helpful
with respect to the cluster of problems. Also, psychotherapy
may be effective in children who have secondary bedwetting
associated with psychological problems. Secondary bedwetting,
which occurs when a child begins wetting after being dry, can be
an indication of psychological problems and it needs professional evaluation. But, as I stressed in the previous chapter, a careful
medical assessment should also be made in case the problem is
not in fact psychological.

Spanking, Shaming, or Scolding Doesn't Help

It is very important that spanking, shaming, or scolding not be
used in handling bedwetting problems. This is true even if the
child is not complying with the program. I do not feel that a

It's very important that spanking, shaming, and scolding not be used in handling the bedwetting problem.

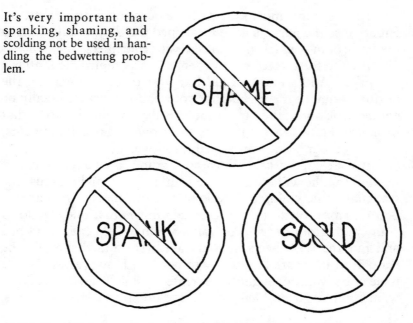

child should be treated until really motivated to become dry, and then, compliance should be less of a problem. One can discuss the relationship between the program and getting dry and review with the child the reason he is being asked to take part in this program.

Q. What should I say to my child if he is not ready for treatment?

A. Usually if a child is wetting at age three or four, he is still going to be in diapers. Mom or Dad has worked with the child to get him dry during the day, and the child has built some self-esteem in terms of accomplishment. Mom is probably praying for the day when she doesn't have to buy diapers anymore, and I'm sure she mentions that to the child, and the child is beginning to understand.

At this stage, most kids do have occasional dry nights, often because the parents have awakened the child to take him to the bathroom—which the child never remembers.

A child feels a tremendous sense of accomplishment after a dry night. And what I would like you to do is focus on the positive—ignore the nights that your child is wet and really be enthusiastic about the times that he is dry. A child is proud that he is dry. He wants his parents to recognize his achievements, and the recognition is an added incentive.

If your child asks, "When am I going to be dry?" you can tell him that he will outgrow the wetting. You might discuss the fact that some children take longer than others, but that if it becomes a problem, there are certain things that one can do. If your child is four or five, you can ask him to help change his bed and put the wet sheets in a certain area, and that might be enough to motivate him to try to get dry. However, the entire issue of bedwetting ought to be treated in a light way. You don't want to create a problem where one doesn't exist.

Q. How can I prevent my child's mattress from getting soaked?

A. Most parents go from having their child wear diapers to using plastic mattress covers and rubber sheets underneath the bottom bed sheet. Children undergoing the bedwetting treatment program should never wear diapers.

Q. What kind of preparations should be made when taking my child on a trip or having him sleep at someone else's house? Should I discuss the bedwetting problem with relatives or friends' parents?

A. Rubber sheets and an extra bottom bed sheet can be sent along to prevent wetting of someone else's bed. Or the child can take his sleeping bag, equipped with its own pad, to sleep in. The problem should be discussed discreetly with relatives or friends' parents so as not to embarrass your child, and perhaps as an added precaution, you could ask the adult to awaken the child during the night to go to the bathroom.

Q. Should my child continue to wear a nighttime diaper?

A. Children aged four or five usually begin to resent wearing a diaper; diapers are very infantilizing. It takes courage on the part of the parents, but I do not favor a child wearing a diaper at age five. You parents at that point have to gut it out, because you are trying to get the child to see himself as growing up, and you don't want to put on that infantilizing diaper that no other children his age wear. So I think parents need to just grit their teeth, put a rubber sheet or pad under the bottom bed sheet, and just do the laundry. I see parents who do have kids wearing diapers, and when I tell the children that they will never wear a diaper again, their reaction is dramatic. The parents take a deep breath and swallow hard at that point. But actually the diaper takes away some of the incentive to get dry because the child doesn't feel the discomfort of the wetness. He has just got a diaper on. You haven't really solved the problem.

Q. If my child is potty trained, should I then expect the child to be dry at night?

A. You should expect your child to be dry during the day before he is able to be dry at night. The one tends to follow the other. Many of the children that I see do have accidents during the day. Their awareness of a full bladder is sometimes weak. Either these kids have their minds elsewhere or they don't get strong enough signals, and thus occasionally they have an accident. It is so important to realize that in the vast majority of cases, daytime accidents and nighttime accidents are not intentional and that the child is devastated by them. You need to handle the problem in a very gentle way.

Q. What is the best time of the year to begin training?

A. It is often harder to get children dry in the summer than it is in the winter. The reasons for this are the change to Daylight Saving Time and the vigorous activities that children tend to get into in the summertime. They are up later and are more tired when they go to bed, and their sleep is deeper. It is a greater challenge to get them to respond to an alarm, or to a parent's prodding, or to a bladder contraction.

When children get dry during the summer, it is usually a very good indicator that they will be dry thereafter. On the other hand, there are some children who get dry during the summer but begin to wet again when school starts because school is a stressor. What it boils down to is that, in general, the more tired children are, whether it is because of physical activity or daytime stress associated with school, the more difficult it will be for them to respond to bladder contractions at night. But if you can guide your child toward the goals set out here—a greater bladder capacity and the ability to respond to a bladder contraction—he ought to be able to stay dry whether he is tired or not.

Q. Does motivation to stop bedwetting vary?

A. Yes. I have kids tell me that there have been times when they were already wet, and cold, and all curled up, and they didn't want to move but they had to go to the bathroom. So they let it rip and they wet on themselves! Now I knew that some kids were doing that, because I did that! So I tell them that I did that, and then I ask if they ever did it, and they sort of smile and say yes. The parents are absolutely astounded. Well, what is the surprise? The child is already wet. Sometimes kids are a little lazy. They know they wet the bed and they know one more time isn't that big a deal. Well obviously, I'm not going to let this happen down the road.

Q. What are some rewards you have found effective in motivating children?

A. I have a verbal contract that says when a child has a certain number of dry or almost-dry nights, he gets a dollar, or maybe two, or we're going to dinner. At the end of the treatment, I give him baseball tickets and the opportunity to treat his dad to a ball game. I'll put my arm around the child and ask him when the last time was that he treated his dad to a ball game. Well, most of them never even thought about that. I say, "How would you like to go up to your dad and say, 'Hey, Dad, how about you and I taking in a game? My treat!'" Not only is there a big smile on the face of the child, but Dad would just love to go to the game with him. To give the child an opportunity to do something mature is part of the success of overcoming this problem. Treating Dad is certainly not something that most children have a chance to do, and they really get a kick out of it.

Q. My child is frequently wet when he returns from playing during the day at his friend's house. How do I train him out of this habit?

A. This is not uncommon. Often a child's attention is on doing, not feeling. He is playing and waits too long to go to the bathroom, so he has an accident. The stream-interruption exercise used in the treatment program will help prevent this daytime wetting. Some parents have found that having their child wear a watch with a timer to remind him to go the the bathroom (e.g., every two hours) is helpful. Younger children usually like the idea of wearing a watch and don't object to this private reminder.

3

Step-by-Step Program

PREPARATION

The treatment program will be a growth experience for your child. This is his problem, and unless he takes responsibility for it, he cannot expect to overcome it. It is important that you become less emotionally involved with the issue, and the only way to do this is to allow your child to take more responsibility for his own treatment. Therefore, your child should be responsible for changing sheets, pajamas, and underwear, although he should not be overwhelmed with this task, especially at the beginning of the program. Some children have already been helping with changing wet clothes, bed sheets, and so on, but if your child has not, it is important to teach him the proper way to remake the bed and to assist him until he is able to take on the responsibility alone. He should be taught, as far as he is able, to fill out the daily log that will be used in the program, and he should be responsible for connecting and disconnecting the wetness alarm that will awaken him at night if he begins to urinate.

Before training begins, talk to your child about the reasons for bedwetting (e.g., small bladder, heredity), his feelings about the problem, and the advantages of being dry. Discuss what treatment steps will be taken and what rewards there will be for

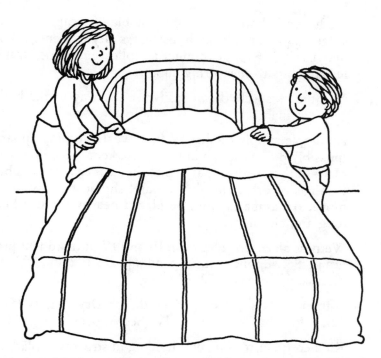

Teach your child how to change the wet bedding and to remake his bed.

progress and for getting dry. Assure him that you will help him, but explain that he will be doing most of the steps himself—he will be in charge—and that the treatment will work, that he will get dry if he does the exercises and follows the other steps.

The treatment program is divided into four phases, and step-by-step instructions will be given for each phase.

Equipment and Supplies You Will Need

- Favorite drinks and snacks for a child to take prior to bladder-capacity measurement.

- Widemouthed measuring cup that holds 16 ounces and is

graduated in half ounces for use in bladder-capacity measurement (available in housewares departments). You may use a different container to collect urine then transfer contents to measuring cup.

- Nightlights so child can easily see the way to the bathroom at night.

- An ample supply of sheets, underwear, sleeping apparel (possibly pillows and blankets also), kept in a convenient place so that changing at night will be as easy as possible. Pajamas or other sleeping apparel should be easy to remove. A hamper should be placed nearby for wet bedding and clothing.

- Wetness alarm for Phases II, III and IV of treatment program. (See supplier list, Appendix pages 102 and 103 and discussion on pages 72-77.)

- Gummed stars (silver and gold) for Dry Nights (Star) Chart for Phases II, III and IV. (See Appendix page 106.)

- Kitchen timer to time withholding in structured bladder-stretching exercise (Phases III and IV).

Q. Should I discuss the treatment with other members of the family?

A. Yes. Once you have decided you are going to start to treat the problem and once your child has said "Look, I really need some help," it is a family problem. There is no question about that, especially when siblings are sharing a bedroom with the child who is being trained. They are involved as well: they are going to be hearing the alarm at night; they are going to have their sleep disturbed; and everyone will be watching the child jump from one foot to the other as he tries to withhold urination as long as he can in the bladder-stretching exercise. It is a family problem, and there needs to be some family understanding of what the child is going to do.

Q. How much responsibility for the treatment can my child take?

A. Ultimately, your child can take responsibility for doing the stream-interruption exercises, reminding you to assist with the paired-association exercises, going to the bathroom at bedtime, and connecting and disconnecting the alarm apparatus. (Obviously, your child cannot be responsible for being awakened after bedtime to go to the bathroom.) Your child can also be responsible for increasing his bladder capacity, but you may have to supervise—you should at least be nearby when your child is measuring the bladder capacity to ensure that the readings are correct. I know of one child who was so highly motivated and so excited about the prospect of receiving a reward for achieving an eight-ounce bladder capacity, that he urinated about four ounces into the toilet and then dipped the cup into the toilet to retrieve eight ounces. He was, however, caught in the act and escaped being punished only because both parents could not stop laughing about the episode.

Preferably, you should continue recording the time that the alarm goes off, and even though you may not be actively involved, be benevolently involved from a distance.

As for the evening snacks and drinks, obviously you cannot monitor them on your own; you need your child's help. Unless you stand right by the refrigerator or pantry door, you will not be completely aware of the voluminous amount of foods and drinks of all varieties that your child consumes.

It's important not to overwhelm the kid at the beginning of the treatment, though. Start off slowly. Let him do the easy things. If you start right off and say, "Well, from now on, you have to watch your diet, you have to do these push-ups, you have to tank up and hold it twice a week, and on top of that, do the laundry every day," you are going to see, somewhere around 5:00 in the afternoon, this kid with a knapsack on his back sneaking out the door heading for the hills.

Q. Why should my child help change the sheets?

A. Oftentimes, parents feel that it is cruel and unusual punishment for their child to have to change the sheets, and I am quite flabbergasted at that response. The response probably occurs more frequently when the child is relatively young, six or seven, but bear in mind that we have waited until the child is old enough to accept that the bedwetting is his own problem. It has been a problem for the parents up until now, and everyone is tired of the laundry, everyone is tired of having to change the sheets. A major aspect of the program is that the child takes responsibility for the bedwetting, and that the child is going to get dry on his own through the various techniques that we are describing.

Making a child change the bed is not a punishment. It should be viewed as assuming responsibility. When the child takes charge of cleaning up, this, if anything, minimizes the embarrassment and ought to enhance his pride: the child is able to handle every aspect of this problem on his own.

One should encourage the child to do this in a positive way rather than implying "They are your sheets, you change them!" Show your child that you are really proud of the way that he is taking responsibility in attacking this problem. Spend some time teaching the child how to operate the washing machine. At age six or seven or eight, this is not too complicated a task: we're dealing with a couple of buttons that have to be pushed. So in the middle of the night if the child wets, the wet things go in the hamper and in the morning they go in the washer.

Q. Why are nightlights important?

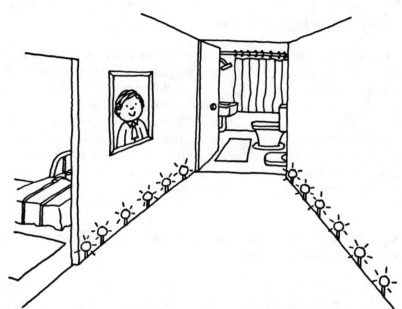

Nightlights are important—they remind your child to get up to go to the bathroom and show him the way.

A. I recommend using nightlights because when kids wake up with signals from a full bladder, we don't want them to go back to sleep. We want them to know that they are to get up and go to the bathroom. They are to do whatever it is that they can do to help themselves have a dry bed.

Now when you are seven years old and you wake up in the middle of the night, and the bathroom is down a dark hall, this can be awfully scary. Unless kids can see where they are going at night, they tend to roll over and go back to sleep. Nightlights are important for these kids to have. You will probably need one in the bathroom and maybe one in the hallway, as well as in the bedroom. I am sure that the satisfaction you have the first time your child actually goes to the bathroom on his own in the middle of the night is well worth the little bit it will cost for the lights.

Q. Should I rearrange my child's room so that his bed is closer to the bedroom door?

A. No, you don't want to change the furniture around so that your child is closer to the door, because many times when kids wake up in the middle of the night, they are confused, they are not fully awake, and their coordination is somewhat limited; they are not functioning at full capacity. So they depend more on their knowledge of the room rather than what actually is there. Keep things as they are. But you do need to make sure there is nothing on the floor that might trip your child. You want to provide a safe pathway for him.

Q. What if my child shares a bedroom, or the same bed with a brother or sister?

A. If your child shares a bed with a brother or sister and wets the bed, the chances are that the two of them aren't getting along very well. Most of the children I see have their own beds, and I would recommend that a child have his own bed if he has this problem, if for nothing else than privacy.

However, I often see children who share a bedroom. It can create some real problems, because there is no question that during the day the memory lingers on and the room has to be aired out. Later in the day, the room may be cold, which leads to complaints if anybody else wants to play in there. We have seen siblings who sleep in bunks, and when it has suddenly started raining on the lower bunk, some rather interesting family situations have arisen.

It would be wonderful if each child could have his own room, for unfortunately, often the roommate may be teasing and really putting pressure on the child who is wetting. One thing you can do, as I explained in Chapter II, is to bring the roommate into the treatment plan. I frequently find that when an older brother or sister is being a pain and taking every opportunity to rub in the bedwetter's failure, having the older child act as a facilitator and sharing the responsibility for the success of the program turns that relationship around.

Phase I

The first phase in the primary bedwetting treatment is mainly a fact-finding period to determine the scope of the problem. In this first two weeks of the program, you will be looking for certain factors that may contribute to wet vs. dry nights, for example, small bladder capacity, irritable bladder, fatigue, or food sensitivity. For this purpose, begin collecting information on the Data Log for Phase I. See the sample log on page 52. A blank form is provided on page 104 in the Appendix. You may use a photocopy of this form or keep the information in a notebook. Have your child begin the exercises described on page 54 to help him get dry.

Begin collecting informa-
tion on the data log.

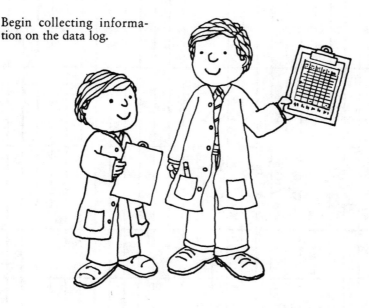

DATA LOG—Phase I

Data log of a six-year-old girl. In this example 5 oz. (the largest amount) is the child's functional bladder capacity. Note that evening snacks and drinks and later bedtimes were probable contributing factors in some bedwetting episodes.

Date	Wet	Dry	Bedtime/ Fell Asleep	Midstream Interrupt	Bladder Stretch	Bladder Capacity (ounces)	# Daytime Bathroom Trips	Evening Snacks and Drinks
2-19		✓	8:50/9:30	✓	✓	2½ oz.	8	Pretzels & cola
2-20		✓	8:00/8:15	✓	✓	5 oz.	10	ice cream
2-21	✓		9:00/9:30	✓	✓		12	
2-22	✓		10:00/10:15	✓			10	chips & soda
2-23		✓	10:00/10:20	✓			12	
2-24	✓		8:00/8:10	✓	✓		9	
2-25		✓	9:00/9:30	✓	✓		9	cookies & milk
2-26	✓		8:00/8:10	✓	✓	4 oz.	8	snacks & drink
2-27	✓		9:30/9:45	✓	✓	2½ oz.	7	snacks & soda
2-28	✓		9:30/9:45	✓	✓		8	
3-1		✓	11:00/11:10	✓	✓		8	
3-2	✓		10:00/10:30	✓	✓		8	snacks & drinks
3-3	✓		9:00/9:15	✓	✓		7	snacks & soda
3-4	✓		9:00/9:15	✓	✓		6	snacks & drink

SAMPLE

Give your child an idea of where things are going to progress. Explain that everything he is about to do, including the stream-interruption and bladder-stretching exercises, is a form of treatment that has a specific track record. It has been tested with other children, and it does work.

Record Keeping. On the Data Log, record the following information:

1. *Wet or dry bed:* Whether child wet or stayed dry at night.

2. *Bedtime and time child actually goes to sleep.* Schedule a regular bedtime; be sure child gets enough sleep. Fatigue increases the depth of sleep. Counsel the child that the more tired he is, the deeper his sleep will be and the less likely he will be aware of the need to go to the bathroom, and so, the greater his chances of wetting the bed.

3. *Midstream-interruption and bladder-stretching exercises.* Indicate that exercises were done. (See instructions on page 54.)

4. *Bladder-capacity measurement:* Number of ounces of urine presented after withholding (see pages 54-56) indicates bladder capacity or at what capacity the child has a full-bladder sensation.

5. *Number of daytime trips to the bathroom:* (five to seven daytime trips is normal.) Frequency of urination may be an indication of bladder irritability or an indication of small bladder capacity. (Note: Frequent urination may also indicate a medical problem and should be checked by a physician.) Discontinue record when number of trips is within normal range.

6. *Evening snacks and drinks:* You may find a relationship between these and the bedwetting. Some foods such as milk, or salty snacks or other foods that may cause your

child to overload on liquids, can contribute to bedwetting. Carbonated and caffeinated drinks, as well as chocolate, have a diuretic effect.

Midstream-interruption (push-up) exercise. This exercise strengthens the outer sphincter muscle, making it easier for the child to hold back urine when there are bladder contractions. It also increases his ability to *control* the outer sphincter muscle—to stop urination using a minimal amout of conscious energy. This is crucial, since the goal is to teach the child to respond to a bladder contraction with an increase in sphincter muscle tone during the night without actually awakening.

How to do it: Each time your child urinates (except when measuring bladder capacity and at bedtime), have him interrupt—stop and start—urination in midstream by tightening (pushing up) the sphincter muscle to stop, then relaxing it to start again. Your child should do this exercise ten times each time he urinates.

Bladder-stretching (withholding) exercise. This exercise increases bladder capacity (the ability of the bladder to hold more urine for a longer time); it also increases the child's awareness of bladder contractions and the sensation of a full bladder.

How to do it: Once a day, have your child delay going to the bathroom for as long as possible. He should tell you when he first feels the need to urinate. Ask him to hold it as long as possible.

Bladder-capacity measurement. In order to determine bladder capacity or at what stage your child feels the need to urinate, measure the number of ounces he urinates after he has held back urine as long as possible.

How to do it: Twice a week, in the morning (Saturday and Sunday are recommended), have your child drink a large caffeinated drink and eat some of his favorite snacks (to encourage him to drink more); ask him to withhold urination for as long as possible. Then have him urinate (without midstream interruption) into a large (16-ounce) wide-mouthed measuring cup (or, if more convenient, use a different container and empty the contents into the measuring cup) and record the number of ounces of urine on the Data Log. (A caffeinated drink is recommended because it will stimulate urine production and assure that urination will happen within a matter of hours. You don't want your child waiting too long and missing other activities.)

Generally, the bladder-capacity data are not consistent, and you should take the highest number of ounces presented during this two-week period as representative of the functional bladder capacity. Most children six to twelve years old have a bladder capacity of about one ounce per year of age; beyond age twelve, capacity is usually fifteen to twenty ounces; for an adult, capacity should measure at least fifteen ounces.

If bladder capacity is below normal, it may be that the child's bladder physically could hold more than the number of ounces given, but once bladder contractions cause serious discomfort, the functional capacity of the bladder has been reached. (As mentioned above, one of the purposes of the bladder-stretching exercise is to improve the child's ability to hold urine comfortably for a longer period of time.)

Bladder-capacity Goals and Rewards

If bladder capacity is below normal, continue the measurement twice a week and set a capacity goal (one ounce per year of age) for your child. Motivate him to achieve the goal by offering a small reward for periodic increases in the measurement. (When I set a goal for a child, I aim high—say six to seven ounces for a six-year-old, ten to twelve ounces for a ten-year-old.)

Studies have shown that bladder capacity can be increased one ounce per month by doing the bladder-stretching exercise. Remember that some children will reach their goal more quickly than others. Often a dramatic increase in bladder capacity is due not to an increased bladder size but to increased muscle tone in the bladder, which results from doing the bladder-stretching exercise and which improves the child's ability to comfortably hold urine longer.

Note that sometimes children stop bedwetting before reaching a normal bladder capacity as a result of following the various steps in the program. That's all right—what we're interested in is the bottom line, the child's getting dry.

If the bladder capacity is normal, no further measurements are necessary; however, your child should continue the bladder-stretching exercise, since its purpose is not only to increase the size of the bladder but also to increase the child's ability to hold urine comfortably for a longer period of time, and to make him more aware of bladder contractions and the sensation of a full bladder. All of these are important assets in staying dry at night. When he continues the bladder-stretching exercise, however, have him use the structured method described on page 91, because this will give him a daily goal to work for.

What to Expect

Although studies have shown that 30 percent of the kids will get dry just by doing the bladder-stretching (withholding) and stream-interruption ("push-up") exercises—and 25 percent of them will respond to motivation alone—most children are still going to be wet after this two-week period, which is mainly a fact-finding stage. Sometimes a child expects instant results, and it is very important for him to realize that bedwetting won't stop right away. This is a scientific preparation. You and the child together are collecting information on the data log, and the child is strengthening his muscles. Later there will be some stronger treatment, but initially he should not expect to get dry.

After two weeks, move to Phase II—see page 69.

Q. How many hours of sleep should my child get?

A. The average sleep requirements are $11\frac{1}{2}$ hours for four-year-olds; 11 hours for five-year-olds; $10\frac{3}{4}$ hours for six-year-olds. By the time children are twelve, they do well with about

9¼ hours of sleep; and by the time they are eighteen, 8¼ hours of sleep is adequate. We find, however, that most of us, including children, are somewhat sleep deprived. Most of us really don't get all the sleep we need. We can get by on far less, but that doesn't necessarily mean that we are functioning maximally on far less. So, I recommend that children six to eight years old get at least 9 to 10 hours of sleep per night.

Your child should make a commitment to getting enough sleep as part of taking responsibility for the treatment, but there should be some flexibility in the schedule for times when there is a special television program or a visit to relatives or friends. It is important for your child to understand, however, that fatigue causes deeper sleep and a greater likelihood that bedwetting will occur.

Q. Why are stream-interruption exercises done so often?

A. Stream-interruption strengthens the outer sphincter muscle, which opens and closes the head of the bladder. I ask chil-

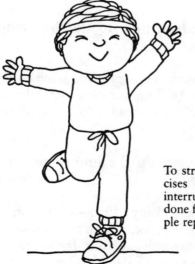

To strengthen muscles, exercises (including midstream-interruption exercise) must be done frequently and in multiple repetitions.

dren how one strengthens a muscle and they all know the answer—by exercising. I ask whether Hulk Hogan got his muscles by doing one push-up once a day. All kids know that one push-up a day just won't do it, that the muscles respond to frequent sets and repetitions of exercise.

Children who wet need to respond to bladder contractions more quickly. They need to respond to a contraction without having to wake up.

So, for a strong response to bladder contractions, I ask kids to stop and start in midstream over and over again, a minimum of ten times per trip to the bathroom. When I describe this, dads usually roll their eyes or wince. Certainly not an easy task for an adult, but it is much easier for the child. I know the kids will come back after two weeks and tell me it got much easier. They are gaining in strength and control of their muscles. Later in the program, even when the children are half asleep in the bathroom, they do their push-ups, or stream-interrruption, exercises automatically; that is the only way they urinate. That's how easy it has become for these kids. But to reach this point requires regular practice.

Q. What's the best time to do the bladder-stretching (withholding) exercise?

A. During the week, an ideal time is when the child comes home from school. Ask him not to run straight to the bathroom as he usually does, but to hold it for as long as he can.

Q. How can I explain the importance of the bladder-stretching exercise?

A. I have two cups in my office—a little cup and a big cup. With a young child, I ask, "Which of these two cups takes longer to fill?" Obviously, it takes longer to fill the big cup. Then I say, "If I give you a small bladder or a big bladder, which would take longer to fill?" Once he understands what a bladder is, it is clear that the big bladder will take longer to fill. "Aha! So if the bladder is big enough, it might take all night to fill!" He understands that. And I say, "If it takes all night and your bladder doesn't fill up until morning, what will happen?" The response is, "I'll be dry."

It is so important for them to understand that one of the goals is to increase the size of the bladder so that it doesn't fill completely during the night. Luckily, six-year-old kids can understand and do realize why they need to work so hard. And they do work hard. It is amazing how these kids can stick to something like this.

Q. How can I make it easier for my child to do the bladder-stretching exercise?

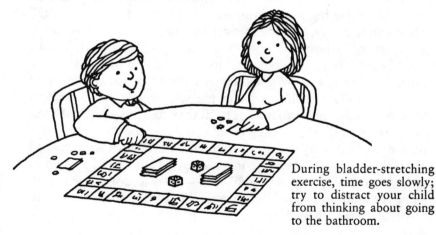

During bladder-stretching exercise, time goes slowly; try to distract your child from thinking about going to the bathroom.

A. When your child first reports a need to go to the bathroom, start paying attention. Try to help distract the child from thinking about the bathroom. If you just ask a kid to hold it and hold it and hold it, time goes painfully slowly. So try to get the child to go outside and play, or do something fun with him. The bladder contraction will pass, but, of course, each succeeding one will feel stronger, until the child will have to go to the bathroom.

Q. Please describe a typical bladder-capacity measurement session.

A. I usually recommend measuring bladder capacity on Saturday and Sunday mornings, assuming that kids don't have basketball, soccer, or some other activity at that time. I ask them to sit down with a sixteen-ounce bottle of cola or soda and drink the whole thing. Have some chips with it, have a party, sit down and watch cartoons and do whatever, and *don't share*. A big smile comes across the kids' faces, and moms look at me like, "I can't believe what this guy is saying. I've been harping on them, *No cola*! He's giving them cola!" Then I ask the kids, "What do you think drinking a cola is going to make you feel like doing?" They will then say, "Going to the bathroom." That is a virtually 100 percent response. They know exactly where I'm at. Then I say "Don't do it, don't do it, don't do it." Without a single exception, no matter where their attention was focused, when I say "Don't do it," they look at me wide-eyed like, "Are you kidding?" I ask them to hold it until they feel the whites of their eyes turning yellow, till they think urine is going to come out of their ears. I jokingly point out to them that throughout recorded time, there has not been one instance of a child who has died of a spontaneously exploding bladder—it just doesn't happen. They are to hold it until they are really dancing from one leg to the other, and when they can't hold it anymore, they are to ask their mom for her favorite measuring cup (which sort of gets a groan from Mom), and then they are to urinate in the measuring cup. That is going to give us an indication of how much their bladder can hold, or at least of how many ounces it can hold comfortably. I also promise a reward if a certain number of ounces is reached.

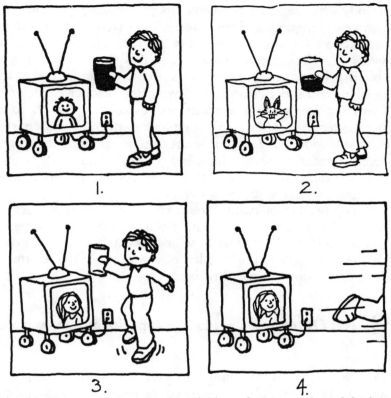

1.

2.

3.

4.

Before bladder-capacity measurement, child eats favorite snacks and drinks a large caffeinated drink—then withholds urination for as long as possible.

Q. Why does urine output vary?

A. Oftentimes a child will give only four ounces after holding back urine for as long as he can, and parents are very frustrated because he didn't give more. Ten minutes later, the same child can go to the bathroom and a copious amount comes out (another four ounces). It's hard for me to imagine that this child, who after three hours produced only four ounces of urine, suddenly had his kidneys go into overdrive, producing urine like nobody's business. More likely, this youngster experienced incomplete empyting, and ten minutes later, with another bladder contraction, he was able to empty out the rest. We are dealing with a bladder-control problem, and this child's experience is not surprising; in fact, it gives us a clue to the nature of the problem and a better idea as to what the bladder capacity is. This child had no idea when he was completely empty. So he just tightened up after eliminating four ounces. He may have a normal bladder capacity but is not completely emptying. If this occurs at bedtime also, it increases the risk of an accident. In a case like this, talk to your child about completely emptying— sometimes kids are just in a hurry.

You need to be really careful about measuring bladder capacity. No one urinates the same amount each time. It depends on the bladder contraction, how uncomfortable you are, possibly the irritability of the bladder, possibly the pH of the urine— there are a lot of factors involved.

Q. Is it OK to measure bladder capacity more than twice a week?

A. No, I don't want you to focus on this too frequently. You need to try not to become overly concerned about it. No matter what I tell parents, though, I still find them measuring bladder capacity every day because they are curious. Don't make this a contest. If you do, you're going to find that your child will have four ounces one time, five ounces the next, three ounces the next, six ounces the next, and two ounces the next, and you will complain that your child is not trying. You should just be interested in the largest amount and some of the variability. In other words, to give an example, when the kid is holding it as long as he can, is he around five ounces each time, with a peak of six or seven, or does he go from two ounces to seven ounces? That will give you some insight into the problem. For example, if your child can sometimes hold nine ounces but feels full and sometimes lets go with only two ounces, either he hasn't always been trying hard to hold back, or he has very strong bladder contractions, which make him feel full. If bladder contractions are a major problem rather than bladder size, he may wet during the night even though he can hold ten to eleven ounces. Also, knowing about a contraction problem helps you understand why a child who may have gone to the bathroom immediately before going to sleep is wet twenty minutes later: The child has an irritable bladder. If bladder contractions are the problem, the withholding exercises may be helpful in teaching him to withstand contractions.

Q. Why should the bladder-capacity measurement be done in the morning?

A. Parents often put on the Data Log, even though I don't ask them for this, the number of ounces of fluid their youngster drank. They say, "He drank sixteen ounces and we only got five ounces back." This is one reason we do the loading in the morning, because what goes in is not what comes out, certainly not at the next urination. It comes out eventually, and if it is put in too late in the day, we all know where it will come out. So that is why this measurement should be done in the morning. Also, you want the child to be able to get on with his day.

Q. What kind of reward is appropriate for reaching a bladder-capacity goal?

A. The deal I make is that when the kids come into my office in two weeks, if they have collected the prescribed amount that we have agreed on, I'll give them a dollar. (Big smile on their faces.) These kids have had dollars before—some have had a lot of money. But no one has ever given them a dollar for urinating. There is something unusual and really enjoyable about this. I'll say, "Has your doctor ever given you a dollar for not urinating or for making a certain number of ounces?" Kids are very enthusiastic and quite confident in their ability to deliver the goods.

Q. Why should my child become more aware of bladder contractions?

A. Children who wet the bed frequently experience more bladder contractions than nonbedwetting children. When bladder contractions occur during very deep sleep, when there is also muscle relaxation, a wet bed results. I often tell children that during the day their bladder at first speaks calmly to them during contractions, saying "I've gotta go to the bathroom." When this happens, say, during school, they know to respond with an outer sphincter muscle closure. In time, they'll be reminded more urgently that they need to go to the bathroom. The bladder speaks with an increasingly loud voice, as bladder contractions become more frequent and stronger. But during sleep, these bladder messages are not heard by some children, and part of the treatment requires an increasing awareness of bladder contractions. I say to the children, "We need to have your bladder scream out to you, *I have to go to the bathroom!*" Being aware of signals from a full bladder may not decrease the frequency of contractions, but it may increase the child's awareness and ability to respond appropriately.

Unfortunately, in many instances, these urgent messages from the bladder occur during the deepest stages of sleep. Studies have shown that auditory awakening thresholds are highest during these stages of sleep, and many parents will attest to the fact that a freight train passing directly through the bedroom six inches from the ear of their sleeping child would not cause the child even to stir. It is not surprising, therefore, that when the bladder screams out for relief, the child, not having heard the recent passing train, does not respond. Part of the training pro-

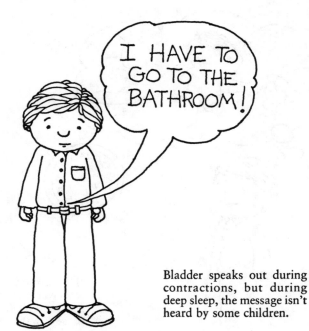

Bladder speaks out during contractions, but during deep sleep, the message isn't heard by some children.

gram, therefore, requires that we attract the child's attention to his poor, contracting bladder. The bladder-stretching exercise accomplishes this goal.

Q. Other than avoiding carbonated and caffeinated drinks, should my child's fluid intake in the evening be restricted?

A. No, I don't believe in fluid restriction. As a former bedwetter whose mother forbade him to drink anything after 7:30 p.m., I have vivid memories of getting my last drink at 7:28 and saying, "I'm not going to drink anything else for the rest of the night,"—and by 7:32 being obsessed with finding or sneaking a drink. I may have had nights where I drank more than I would have only because someone said to me, "You can't have anything to drink after 7:30." It doesn't work.

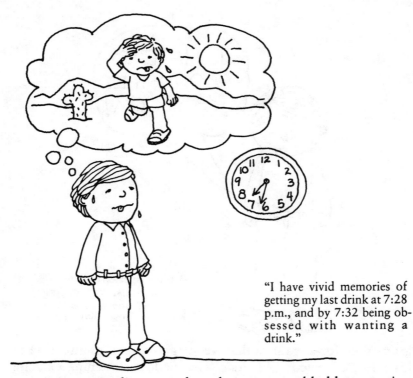

"I have vivid memories of getting my last drink at 7:28 p.m., and by 7:32 being obsessed with wanting a drink."

As parents discover when they measure bladder capacity, what goes in doesn't come out immediately, and what goes in is not necessarily reflected in the next urination. I have yet to have a parent report that fluid restriction is effective. It is just something to try. It seems logical: if he doesn't drink, he won't urinate. It is logical, but that isn't the way it works. However, your child shouldn't *overload* on fluids in the evening.

Q. What's the connection between evening snacks and bedwetting?

A. Salty foods can be a problem. I often find that youngsters are snacking on potato chips, pretzels, cheese curls—you name it. Everything seems to have a little salt or seasoning on it. I have

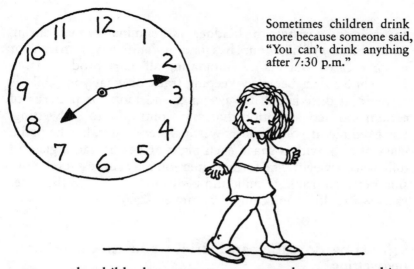

Sometimes children drink more because someone said, "You can't drink anything after 7:30 p.m."

yet to see the child who eats popcorn, pretzels, or potato chips and doesn't wash all of it down with some kind of drink.

As I've said, I don't believe in fluid restriction, but let's be reasonable: loading up with fluids is not going to make things easier either.

Children have to make some choices. A child working in this program is supposed to have recognized that the bedwetting is a problem he wants to solve. A total sacrifice of snacks isn't requested, just modification of what is consumed in the evening, because salty foods make a child thirsty and loading up with fluids right before bedtime doesn't make a lot of sense, especially in a kid who wets three and four times a night. So, the child has to be prepared to make a small sacrifice. Mom or Dad can make it easier by having nonsalty food available as munchies in the evening.

Q. Can food allergies contribute to bedwetting?

A. Yes, as mentioned earlier, food allergies may cause the bladder to become more irritable, and I have found that milk in particular may irritate the bladder. Just eliminating milk during dinner or the evening hours has made a significant improvement in some cases. But before eliminating all dairy products from your child's diet, begin by keeping track of what your child is eating and drinking in the evening, and look for patterns of certain food consumption that may contribute to bedwetting. For example, if your child is wetting every night, has he had a glass of milk with a snack each night or has he had a glass of milk once a week? The former situation may suggest a relationship between drinking milk and bedwetting, while in the latter case, withholding milk might be unnecessary.

Q. How do caffeinated drinks and chocolate affect bedwetting?

A. Watch out for the following three compounds: caffeine, theophylline, and theobromine, which are part of a group of chemicals called methylxanthines. Methylxanthines have a number of properties in common, one of which is that they all act as a diuretic—they make you urinate. Caffeine is in cola and coffee, of course. Theophylline is usually found in tea, and theobromine is in chocolate.

I ask kids, "Which would you rather have—a theobromine chocolate sundae right before bed or a dry bed?" (The answer is supposed to be "a dry bed.")

Now, chocolate is tempting, and most of us, when confronted with sin, if it's right there, find it very, very tough to deny ourselves. But it is very important for your child to avoid chocolate.

However, every rule is made to be broken, and I don't know that having a scoop of chocolate ice cream occasionally is necessarily going to make much difference. After all, bedwetting is not a medical emergency. We want your child motivated and we want him to understand and we want him to follow the rules. But let's say he has a friend staying over or he is going to

Grandma's house and everybody else is eating Grandma's chocolate cake. I think it is cruel and unusual punishment not to give
your child some, unless he decides on his own to abstain.

The rules here are guidelines, and guidelines have to have
some flexibility. The worst thing that is going to happen is that
your child will have another wet night. You've been there
before. It's not anything to get overly worked up about.

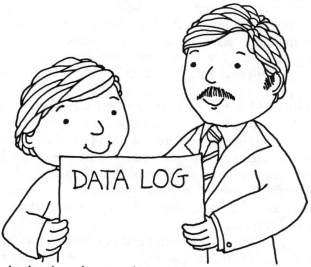

Review the data log—focus on the positive.

Phase II

As you go into the second phase of the treatment, focus on
the positive. For example, ask your child, "Are you doing your
push-ups (stream-interruption exercises) and have they gotten
easier to do?" If your child has been doing these exercises and
they have gotten easier, that means the outer sphincter muscle is
getting stronger, and that's terrific. Talk about how proud you
are that he has been doing the push-ups and the bladder-stretching exercises. Tell him that he has to work at them every day—
that's the way he's going to beat the bedwetting problem.

Review Data Log

You have information on whether your child was wet or dry
and on what time he went to bed. You know how many times
he went to the bathroom each day and what he was eating and
drinking in the evening. If your child started by going to the
bathroom eight or ten times a day and you see a gradual decrease, this tells you that the bladder exercises are almost certainly either increasing the size of the bladder or helping him to
hold back urination longer. And in most cases, you will know
bladder capacity is actually increasing because your measurements will show it. These improvements are wonderful. Even
though your child may still wet, there is something positive—he
is making progress.

If your child is having both dry and wet nights, look for
patterns. What time he went to bed. What he was eating in the
evening. He ate this, he wet here. He didn't eat this, he was dry.
Three or four nights he went to bed late; the next night he was
exhausted, and even though he went to bed on time, that night
he wet. The patterns aren't always crystal clear, but there will be
some indication of the relationship between the child's activities
and diet and the bedwetting.

If bladder-capacity measurement is below the average for
your child's age, you can conclude that either he has a small
bladder capacity or he feels unusually uncomfortable long
before full bladder capacity is reached. It doesn't matter if the
child's bladder holds a hundred ounces; if he's horribly uncomfortable at four ounces, four ounces is the capacity you're dealing with. (As mentioned previously, one of the purposes of the
bladder-stretching exercise is to increase the child's ability to
hold urine comfortably for a longer period of time.) Continue to
set periodic goals for increases in bladder-capacity measurement
and reward your child for reaching the goals.

Continue the following:

DATA LOG—Phase II

Excerpt from data log of six-year-old boy responding regularly to the wetness alarm: earning silver stars. Note increase in bladder capacity measurement and decrease in number of wetting episodes. Depending on age, physical maturity and other individual differences of each child, there will be many variations on this example.

Date	Wet	Dry	Bedtime/ Fell Asleep	Wetting Time (alarm sounded) *small wet spot	Exercises Done: Midstream Interrupt/PAX	Exercises Done: Bladder Stretch	Bladder Capacity (ounces)	# Daytime Bathroom Trips
9-1	✓		10:15/10:30	5:00*	✓	✓		8
9-2	✓		4:30/9:40	10:50*-12:00*-1:25*	✓	✓		8
9-3		✓	8:00/9:00	—		✓		7
9-4	✓		8:10/8:30	11:30*	✓	✓	5 oz.	8
9-5	✓		9:15/9:25	11:52-*-2:00*	✓	✓	5 oz.	7
9-6		✓	9:00/9:15	—	✓	✓		8
9-7	✓		8:45/9:00	11:45*	✓	✓		8
9-8	✓		8:15/8:30	10:00*-4:00*	✓	✓		7
9-9		✓	8:30/8:40	—	✓	✓		8
9-10	✓		8:30/8:45	9:45-3:00/no star	✓	✓		8
9-11	✓		8:30/8:45	? star	✓	✓	5½ oz.	9
9-12	✓		8:45/9:00	10:00-5:30/no star	✓	✓	6 oz.	8
9-13	✓		8:15/8:30	11:50*	✓	✓		7
9-14		✓	8:30/8:40		✓	✓		8
9-15	✓		8:20/8:36	11:30*	✓	✓		8
9-16	✓		8:20/8:30	1:00*	✓	✓		8
9-17	✓		8:00/8:20	1:30*	✓	✓		8
9-18	✓		10:30/10:45	?*	✓	✓		8
9-19	✓		8:00/8:30	1:05*	✓	✓		7
9-20	✓		8:30/8:45	12:30 no star	✓	✓	5 oz.	7
4-21	✓		9:00/9:30	1:15*	✓	✓	5½ oz.	7
9-22	✓		8:00/8:15	1:55**	✓	✓		8
9-23		✓	8:10/8:30	—	✓	✓		8
9-24		✓	8:45/9:00		✓	✓		7
9-25	✓		8:00/8:25	1:05*	✓	✓		7
9-26	✓		8:35/8:45	3:00*	✓	✓		8
9-27	✓		10:00/10:15	2:00*	✓	✓		7
9-28	✓		8:30/8:45	2:20*	✓	✓		7
9-29		✓	8:30/8:40	—	✓	✓		7

SAMPLE

- Data Log. See sample Phase II completed log on page 71. A blank form is provided on page 105 in Appendix. (Note space for recording times the wetness alarm goes off; also see page 79.) You may use photocopies of this form or keep the information in a notebook.

- Midstream-interruption (push-up) exercise ten times each urination (see page 54).

- Bladder-stretching (withholding) exercise once daily (see page 54); if bladder capacity is normal, use structured method (see page 91).

- Bladder-capacity measurement twice a week (see pages 54-56); discontinue when normal capacity has been reached.

- Monitoring child's evening snacks and drinks (see pages 53-54); written record may be discontinued. (If there is a problem you want to continue following, a record can be kept on a separate sheet of paper.)

At this time you should introduce the wetness alarm, begin conditioning (paired-association or PAX) exercises to help the child respond to the alarm, and set up a nighttime training routine (see pages 79-80). Your child should be taking as much responsibility as possible for the treatment, such as changing sheets, keeping the data log and doing the exercises.

It is important to note that the wetness alarm is a vital part of the treatment. In fact, it is 65 percent effective in stopping bedwetting even if nothing else is done. And usually, even before the child stays dry all night, there will be a dramatic improvement in the problem, such as a decrease in the size of the wet spots in the bed.

Wetness Alarm—How It Works

The bedwetting alarm systems consist of a sensor that is at-

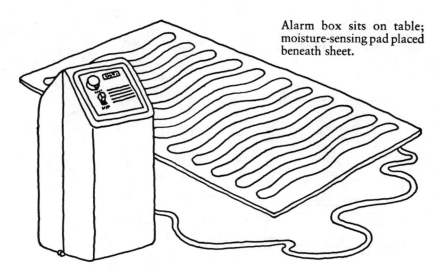

Alarm box sits on table; moisture-sensing pad placed beneath sheet.

tached to an alarm and a battery. The circuit is fluid-activated. The simplest systems consist of a sensor pad which is placed beneath the sheet. When the sheet becomes wet, a harmless circuit is formed and the alarm sounds. In other systems small sensors connected to the alarm are placed in the underpants or clipped to them, and when the child begins to wet, the moisture activates the alarm. The advantage of these latter systems is that the alarm is triggered more quickly, giving the child the opportunity to wake up before the bed is completely soaked. The alarms vary in the type and intensity of the sound they emit and the method by which they are kept in place. Some are fastened to a shoulder patch or to the wrist; some are contained in a waistband. But essentially the mechanisms are identical.

The alarms that are on the market today are extremely safe. One of the things that I have the kids do is hold the alarm in their hands and let it buzz. There may be a vibration, but there is no painful sensation.

In using these devices, the child learns to respond to the alarm by stopping urination. There should be a spontaneous tightening of the outer sphincter muscle, causing the child to

Alarm attached to pajama
collar or shoulder; mois-
ture-sensing pad worn in
underpants.

Buzzer attached to pajama
shoulder; moisture-sensing
strip attached to outside of
underpants.

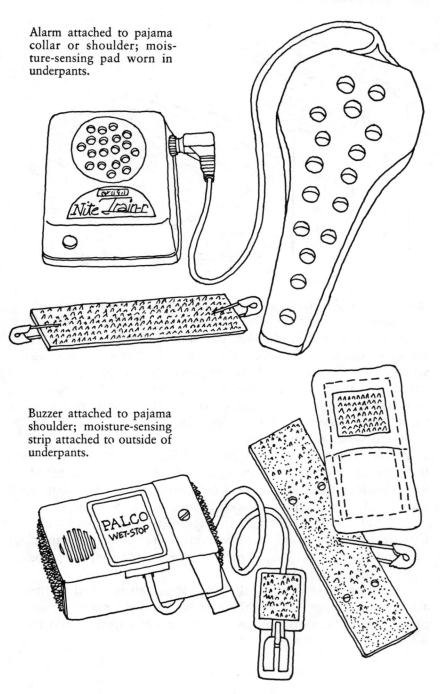

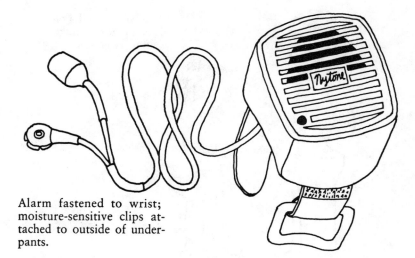

Alarm fastened to wrist; moisture-sensitive clips attached to outside of underpants.

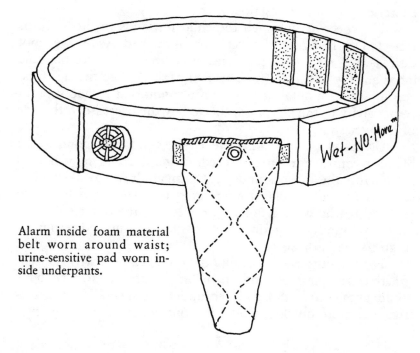

Alarm inside foam material belt worn around waist; urine-sensitive pad worn inside underpants.

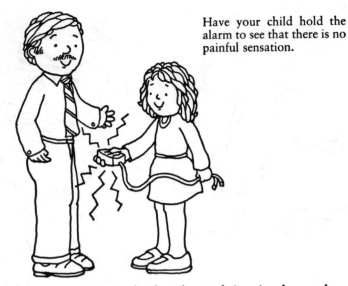

Have your child hold the alarm to see that there is no painful sensation.

stop in midstream (just as he has been doing in the push-up exercises previously described).

The speed with which the child responds to the alarm is reflected in the size of the wet spot on the bed. As the wet spot decreases in size, it is quite clear that the child is responding more quickly to the alarm. This is the critical step that must be accomplished in obtaining successful conditioning, that is, rapid responsivity to the alarm as reflected by the decrease in the size of the wet spot.

Ultimately, the goal is to teach the child to respond to the bladder contractions that precede urination and to wake up even before the alarm sounds, just as an adult will awaken a few seconds before the alarm clock goes off. The child learns to respond to the contractions by tightening the outer sphincter muscle to prevent urination, and possibly waking and getting up to go to the bathroom.

For the purpose of conditioning, one can see why the sensors that fit right in the underpants or are attached to them have an advantage over those placed under the sheet. The alarm is triggered more quickly, while the contraction is still ongoing.

The conditioning devices themselves have a 65 to 70 percent success rate according to the literature, and in most cases, if the child does nothing else other than wear the device, he has a two-thirds chance of ultimately achieving dryness. I feel, however, that the midstream-interruption and bladder-stretching exercises enhance the effectiveness of the alarm for two main reasons. The alarm often only partially awakens the child, causing confusion. And if the child cannot tighten the outer sphincter until he is fully awake, that is usually too late. The exercises help the child to gain excellent control of the outer sphincter muscle and increase bladder capacity and awareness of bladder contractions.

Occasionally I see conflicts between my experience with the alarm systems and that claimed by the manufacturers. Often the manufacturers cite a much higher degree of responsivity to the system than I have found; and frequently they assert that no stream-interruption or bladder-stretching exercises are needed, nor awakenings for trips to the bathroom. It is quite possible that the type of patient that I see in the clinic is more resistant to treatment than those seen by the manufacturers. However, I feel that my recommendations enhance the likelihood of success.

For information on where to buy wetness alarms, see Appendix, pages 102 and 103.

Introduce Wetness-activated Alarm

Discuss the alarm with your child. Show him how it works; assist him in putting it on, in connecting and disconnecting it. Explain that he will wear the alarm nightly to help him stop wetting the bed. When he hears the alarm, it will be his job to stop urinating and turn it off. Tell him that you will help him wake up when the alarm goes off and that you will go with him to the bathroom. Only your child should disconnect the alarm to ensure that he does reach some level of alertness and is aware of what is going on. I tell children that Mom and Dad have the right to awaken them in any way they choose—screaming, stomping, etc.—but that the one thing they are not allowed to do is turn off the alarm. Only the child can turn the alarm off because it belongs to him.

It is important that your child wear the alarm every night. Conditioning the child to awaken or respond to bladder sensations requires regular reinforcement. If the alarm doesn't go off consistently when the child wets, it's going to take that much longer for him to learn not to wet. So it's important that you be consistent here and that the child try to wear the alarm every night.

Introduce the Paired-Association Exercise (PAX)

In addition to the stream-interruption (push-up) exercises your child is doing at each urination to strengthen the outer sphincter muscle and increase his ability to respond to a bladder contraction, next you need to help your child respond very, very quickly when the alarm goes off. By doing a conditioning exercise called paired association, or PAX, he will learn to respond with a push-up almost reflexively whenever the alarm goes off, and there will be some carry-over into the night. This exercise can reduce the bedwetting treatment time by as much as two weeks. So, explain to your child that this exercise will help him stop wetting and shorten the time necessary to achieve dryness.

How to do it: Once a day, preferably at the same time each day, have your child go to the bathroom accompanied by one or both parents. Bring the wetness alarm and either stand outside the door or in the bathroom with your back to the child. Have him begin to urinate in the toilet, and shortly after urination begins, manually trigger the alarm. It is the child's job to stop in midstream as quickly as possible in response to the alarm. Tell him not to anticipate the alarm, and then trigger it at variable intervals (try to do it at least three times), so that the child learns to respond reflexively to the alarm by stopping urination in midstream. (Note on data log that exercise has been done.) Discontinue the exercise when the child is regularly responding to the alarm at night with just a small wet spot.

Nighttime Training Routine

1. *Have your child go to the bathroom precisely at bedtime, without doing push-ups.* He should completely empty the bladder.

2. *At bedtime have your child wear the alarm.* Assist him in the correct placement and connecting of the alarm apparatus according to the manufacturer's instructions. Remind him that when the alarm goes off, he is to stop urinating, disconnect the alarm, and go to the bathroom to finish urinating. Tell him that you will help him wake up and go with him to the bathroom, but that only he is to disconnect the alarm (so that he is aware of what is happening).

3. *Awaken your child one hour after bedtime and take him to the bathroom.* This will help delay wetting to a later time of night when sleep is lighter and your child's chances of hearing and responding to the alarm are greater. Have your child disconnect the alarm and take him to the bathroom. No push-ups need to be done at this time, but many children are so used to doing them that they will do them even when half asleep. When your child is back in bed, help him reconnect the alarm.

4. *When the alarm goes off,* assist your child in waking up—but only he should disconnect the alarm. Guide him to the bathroom and help him return to the bedroom. Then record on the Data Log the time the alarm went off. Your child should change his pajamas, underpants, and sheets and place them in the laundry hamper. When he is back in bed, help him reconnect the alarm. Repeat the procedure as necessary.

5. *Have your child begin keeping a Dry Nights ("Star") Chart.* (See sample completed chart on page 80.) A blank chart is provided in the Appendix, page 106. You

DRY NIGHTS MONTH OF: SEPTEMBER						
SUNDAY	MONDAY	TUESDAY	WEDNESDAY	THURSDAY	FRIDAY	SATURDAY
1 silver	2 silver	3 gold	4 silver	5 silver	6 gold	7 silver
8 silver	9 gold	10 no star	11 no star	12 no star	13 silver	14 gold
15 silver	16 silver	17 silver	18 silver	19 silver	20 no star	21 silver
22 silver	23 gold	24 gold	25 silver	26 silver	27 silver	28 silver
29 gold	30 silver					

Silver star: Awakened by alarm—a small wet spot
Gold star: Stayed dry all night

Chart corresponds to sample Phase II data log, page 71.

may use photocopies of this chart to record dry nights or you may want to make a larger calendar chart on poster paper. Post the chart near your child's bed so it will be convenient for affixing the stars.

Usually within a matter of weeks, a child is responding to the alarm and has a noticeably smaller wet spot on the sheet. Check your child's bed and award a silver star for a small wet spot, a gold star for a dry night, or no star for a large wet spot. (A different method may be used for an older child if stars are not appropriate.) Offer a small reward for a consecutive number of silver or gold stars. The chart is a source of pride for the child and is something he can show to grandparents or other family members.

What to Expect

You should see one or more indications of progress. Specifically, the number of times that the child goes to the bathroom during the day usually tends to decrease as bladder stretching increases the capacity of the bladder. The number of ounces the child can withhold tends to increase. His push-ups become easier. The length of time that the child can withhold urination tends to increase. The alarm tends to go off increasingly later during the night and the number of bedwetting events during the course of the night tends to decrease. The size of the wet spot tends to get smaller as he learns to respond to the alarm and the number of dry nights tends to increase.

With all of these potential improvements at each step in the program, you should find *some* sign that your child is making progress, and you can praise and reward him at that point.

If your child isn't responding to the treatment, rather than thinking that the overall treatment isn't working, try to find out what *part* of the treatment isn't effective. Be sure that your child is getting enough sleep and isn't overtired from too much activity during the day. Be sure that he is doing the bladder-stretching exercise to help increase bladder capacity and make him more aware of bladder contractions and the feeling of a full bladder. Encourage him to do the stream-interruption (push-up) exercise to strengthen the outer sphincter muscle and to help him respond to bladder contractions, and the paired-association exercise to help him respond to the alarm. It's important to know where the battle lines are so that your child doesn't feel like he's failing. Instead, he needs to understand what part of the treatment he has to work on.

Usually, by the end of approximately four weeks, the child begins to earn silver stars (for a smaller wet spot). Occasionally, a child earns a series of gold stars (for a dry bed) within the first few days of wearing the alarm. I tell parents not to get too excited about this. I tell them that I am sure they are delighted, but that the wetting problem is not yet solved. The key is first getting silver stars; this indicates a response to the alarm, and the silver stars will eventually give way to gold. Bear in mind that on nights when the alarm does not go off, no conditioning is taking place. So if your child has five or six dry nights in a row, no alarm has been sounding, and no conditioning occurs. On the other hand, when your child responds to the alarm with silver stars, and then we see a series of dry nights, this reflects true conditioning and true learning.

Also, bear in mind that this type of program involves a two-steps-forward, one-step-back type of progress because when conditioning is not taking place, *deconditioning* occurs. An example of this would be if you were to practice reciting a list of words; after a certain number of trials, the ability to recall those words is greatly enhanced, but then if you stop practicing, you forget. However, a fairly short period of review may be all that's required to recover the memory that was lost. Similarly, as a child has longer and longer periods of dryness (when the alarm doesn't sound), there may be lapses—occasional series of nights of wetness—even though progress is really being made.

If your child does not respond to the alarm at all, it is really important to help and encourage him to wake up. Shake him or talk to him to get him to turn off the alarm. It may be necessary to stay in the same room with your child for awhile until he gets the idea. It may also be necessary to awaken the child to go to the bathroom an hour and a half after bedtime rather than an hour after bedtime (again, to postpone wetting so the alarm will go off later, when sleep is lighter, and the child will be more likely to respond to it). However, if your child is wetting three and four times a night, this is not going to help much. For example, if he is normally wetting at 11:30 p.m., 3:00 a.m., and then 5:00 a.m., waking him an hour and a half after bedtime means you still will have the alarm going off at 3:00 a.m. and 5:00 a.m. This is discouraging, but if you can get the child to respond to some of the wetting and alarms, my experience suggests that there will be a transferrence and the child will start responding to all of the signals. What you will probably see is a response first to the last wet-and-alarm signal, and then gradually a decrease in the number of times the child wets per night. The pattern of wetness will change. You may still have an 11:00 p.m. or 11:30 p.m. wetting that leaves the child really wet, but in the rest of the mishaps, the wets are quite small. That's important, and that is a very, very big improvement. When your child is responding to the alarm in this way, move the awakening time from an hour and a half to one hour after bedtime.

Sometimes, when the child sleeps through the alarm regularly right from the beginning or learns to respond to an alarm but eventually begins to sleep through it, it's necessary to try a different alarm. It is not uncommon to use two or three types of alarms within one schedule of treatment—different children react to different types of noises.

It is important, however, to recognize where the problem lies. If your child does not respond to the alarm, and if it is very difficult to arouse him by touching or shaking him, depth of sleep is the basic problem. Try to be sure your child gets more sleep. And be sure to awaken him for a trip to the bathroom after bedtime, as mentioned above. Thus, the alarm will not be triggered until later at night, when sleep becomes lighter.

When your child is showing a good response to the alarm— earning silver stars regularly—move on to Phase III. See page 88.

Q. What if my child doesn't make the bladder measurement goal?

A. Sometimes children fail to make the goal and don't earn anything. What I often do then is say to them, "Well, you didn't make it, but if you make it next week, why don't you call me because I'd love to hear that and I will send you a dollar in the mail." I may get a phone call on a Saturday morning in the office or a Saturday afternoon at home, and this little high-pitched voice will say, "Dr. Scharf, this is Scott!" I think, "Oh, my God, I have eight Scotts in the clinic—who is Scott?"

"Dr. Scharf, I made seven ounces!"

"Well, that's terrific! I'll put your dollar in the mail."

I don't know if seven ounces is really an improvement for Scott, or if he is pulling the wool over my eyes. I don't have the chart in front of me. But you've got to be enthusiastic. The children call because this is something that means a lot to them. So, sometimes you need to reset goals and encourage your child to reach them.

Q. How can I help my child accept using the alarm?

A. I recommend that the alarm be introduced as a tool that can eventually be used as a toy. I frequently tell children that this alarm (depending on its type) can be worn when skating or biking, and used like a bell. Or, they can eventually hang the alarm outside their door so that anyone wanting to enter will have to ring first. The children tend to think this is a lot of fun and then are less frightened by the alarm.

You certainly should help your child to attach the alarm, showing him what happens when it goes off, and have him disconnect it.

Q. Don't children get upset when they're awakened by the alarm?

A. Some children do get quite disturbed when the alarm goes off during the night, and parents have told me they felt this was cruel and unusual punishment for something as insignificant as bedwetting.

In fact, I have known parents who woke up confused, turning off their own alarm clocks, looking for the smoke detector, and so on. But when a child wakes up in the morning dry for the first time, the trade-off is really quite remarkable and the child feels generally quite satisfied.

The crying that may occur on the first night or two with the alarm is no different from the crying that occurs when parents awaken the child to take him to the bathroom. These trips are generally accompanied by confusion, crying, crabbiness, and so on. This is natural. And for most children there are no bad effects from being awakened by either parents or the alarm.

Q. Why should I record the time the alarm goes off?

A. This gives you some indication as to whether or not increasing bladder capacity is helping the child get over the problem, and it very often does. You will notice that as bladder capacity increases, the time the alarm goes off becomes later. Also, recording the times the alarm sounds gives you an idea of the scope of the problem. Quite frequently a child is wetting three and four times a night, and although parents had suspected this was happening, seeing the times recorded makes them realize the extent of the problem and that this is not something that their child is doing intentionally. If you have a situation like this, you need to have a little patience. If your records show that your child has cut back on wetting from four times a night to once a night, that is a tremendous improvement—but a wet bed is still the end result every morning, and you still have to dry your child out.

Q. What can I do to increase the chances that my child will hear the alarm?

A. One method is to be sure to follow the instruction to wake up your child an hour after bedtime. This will delay wetting and consequent alarm sounding to a later part of the night, when sleep is lighter.

Also, see to it that your child is not overly tired. So often I find that children who wet the bed are going to bed too late at night, and the more tired they are, the deeper they sleep. Being overtired is almost a guarantee of a wet bed.

Q. Is there any way I can adjust the alarm so my child will hear it more readily?

A. I have tried all kinds of techniques, including having Mom make a headband from a cut-up pair of pantyhose so the child can wear the alarm at ear level. Often this is quite helpful.

Q. What if my child disconnects the alarm but doesn't get up to go to the bathroom?

A. Sometimes when that happens, the child is dry for the rest of the night or all you find is a small wet spot. Other times you find a child who is soaking wet. Parents think, "Well, he wet and he just took the alarm off." But what may have happened is that the child did respond to the alarm, woke up partially, stopped wetting, and then went back to sleep. And then the next time he had a bladder contraction, he completely emptied his bladder. This is why when the alarm goes off, Mom or Dad should be there—at least at the beginning—to help the child, because oftentimes, the child is doing far better than his parents realize. Ultimately the aim is to get your child to be able to hold it through the night. But in the meantime, you should look for more episodes in which the child wakes up and wants to go to the bathroom. Even if he needs a parent's help to get there, this is a very positive sign. That the child is responding in a new way is another indication that he is making progress.

Q. What does the size of the wet spot on the child's bed indicate?

A. The idea is for the child to respond to the alarm as quickly as possible, and the way we know that this has occurred is when the wet spot has become increasingly smaller. Eventually, when the child is responding regularly to the alarm, the wet spot often is on the underwear only. With that, the child has very little to do other than changing his underwear. Everybody then has a good feeling. Some children at this point are quite satisfied and no longer highly motivated. After all, Mom and Dad are much happier. The child is turning off the alarm so quickly that the parents don't hear it and don't have to get up to help him. In most cases, once the child is responding to the alarm and once the size of the wet spot is small, success is right around the corner. It's obvious that the alarm has helped the child learn to respond quickly to bladder contractions. In fact, a small wet spot means he is responding only a second or two late. However, he should continue to wear the alarm until the wet spots no longer appear.

Q. What do you consider a small wet spot?

A. If the child can continue wetting in the bathroom, he has left only a small wet spot on the bed. A spot limited to the underwear or slightly wetting the bed is a small spot.

Q. How long will I have to continue waking my child after bedtime?

A. The child is not going to be awakened by his Mom or Dad forever. I reassure parents that this is not something that is going to be a permanent situation. I often tell kids that I don't want Mom or Dad to be coming into their room every night all the way up until they get married. Once your child is responding to the alarm, you are gradually pulled out of the picture. Instructions are given in the treatment program for a gradual phasing out of the waking process.

Phase III

As you begin this third phase, it is assumed that your child is beginning to respond to the treatment, that is, regularly earning silver stars for a small wet spot. At this time, it is important to review the progress he has made and to make some modifications in the treatment plan.

Review Data Log and Dry Nights (Star) Chart

The Phase II Data Log and Star Chart will indicate how well your child is responding to the alarm. When you look at the wetting times on the Data Log (when the alarm goes off), you will often see a change there. The alarm may be going off later and the number of times the child wets tends to decrease. Also, the size of the wet spot tends to get smaller and the number of dry nights tend to increase. You will probably see an increase in bladder capacity and a decrease in the number of daytime bathroom trips.

There are so many opportunities here to show improvement, and nothing motivates like success—success breeds success. Look for things that your child can feel good about, signs that he is coming closer to being dry.

When silver or gold stars appear on the Star chart, praise your child and let him know that he is doing it on his own. Reward him for goals reached.

Continue the following:

- Data Log and Dry Nights (Star) chart. See Phase III samples on pages 89 and 90. (Blank forms provided in the Appendix, pages 106 and 107.)

- Midstream-interruption (push-up) exercise ten times each urination (see page 54).

- Bladder-stretching (withholding) exercise once daily (see page 54); *introduce structured technique as indicated on page 91.*

DATA LOG—Phase III

Excerpt from data log of nine-year-old boy consistently responding to the wetness alarm—earning silver stars for a small wet spot—then having an increasing number of dry nights—earning gold stars. Note that wetting is occurring quite late at night in the majority of cases as bladder capacity and withholding time increase. When the wetting occurs earlier at night, it tends to happen when the child is overly tired. There will be many variations on this example, depending on the age, physical maturity and other individual differences in each child.

Date	Wet	Dry	Bedtime/ Fell Asleep	Wetting Time (alarm sounded) *small wet spot	Exercises Done: Midstream Interrupt	Bladder Stretch (minutes held)	Bladder Capacity (ounces)	# Daytime Bathroom Trips
5-28	✓		9:40/9:55	3:25*	✓	90	7½ oz. normal	5
5-29	✓		8:40/8:50	4:50 no star	✓	91	capacity	4
5-30	✓		9:20/9:30	5:36*	✓		reached	5 (within
5-31	✓		8:50/9:05	1:16*	✓			normal
6-1	✓		9:00/9:15	1:30 star	✓	98		range)
6-2		✓	10:10/10:36	—				
6-3	✓		9:00/9:10	1:30-2:55 star no star				
6-4		✓	9:00/9:10	—				
6-5		✓	9:05/9:15	—				
6-6		✓	8:45/9:00	—				
6-7	✓		9:00/9:10	2:55*	✓			
6-8		✓	11:00/11:10	—	✓			
6-9	✓		9:00/9:10	6:05*	✓	99		
6-10		✓	9:10/9:30	—	✓			
6-11			9:30/9:40	—	✓			
6-12	✓		9:40/9:45	4:07*	✓			
6-13	✓		10:00/10:10	4:55*	✓			
6-14		✓	10:00/10:10	—	✓	108		
6-15		✓	11:30/11:40	—	✓			
6-16		✓	12:30/12:40	—	✓			
6-17		✓	11:10/11:20	—	✓	109		
6-18	✓		9:30/9:40	12:30*	✓			
6-19		✓	10:30/10:40	—	✓	120		
6-20		✓	9:30/9:40	—	✓	↑		
6-21			9:00/9:15	—	✓	new records		
6-22			9:30/9:40	—	✓			
6-23			10:00/10:10	—	✓			
6-24		✓	10:20/10:30	—	✓			
6-25		✓	9:00/9:10	—	✓			

SAMPLE

DRY NIGHTS MONTH OF: MAY-JUNE						
SUNDAY	MONDAY	TUESDAY	WEDNESDAY	THURSDAY	FRIDAY	SATURDAY
			28 silver	29 —	30 silver	31 silver
June 1 —	2 gold	3 —	4 gold	5 gold	6 gold	7 silver
8 gold	9 silver	10 gold	11 gold	12 silver	13 silver	14 gold
15 gold	16 gold	17 gold	18 silver	19 gold	20 gold	21 gold
22 gold	23 gold	24 gold	25 gold	26 gold		

Silver star: Awakened by alarm—a small wet spot
Gold star: Stayed dry all night

Chart corresponds to sample Phase III data log, page 89.

- Bladder-capacity measurement twice a week (see pages 54-56); *discontinue when normal capacity is reached.*

- Monitoring child's evening snacks and drinks (see pages 53-54); written record not required.

- Child's trip to bathroom at bedtime (no push-ups at this time).

- Nightly alarm use (see pages 77-78 and 79).

- Awakening child after bedtime to go to bathroom—*but adjust time as indicated below.*

Adjust awakening time. If your child is responding to the alarm and earning silver stars consistently (two-thirds of the time), awaken him half an hour instead of an hour after bedtime to go to the bathroom. Even with this earlier awakening, it is hoped that the child will still reflexively respond to the alarm and earn a silver star. If silver stars continue to be earned, eliminate awakening completely. The goal is to have your child awaken on his own.

Introduce some structure to the bladder-stretching exercise (see page 54). Each day your child should attempt to increase the length of time that he can withhold urination. The reason it is important to set this goal is that this exercise becomes rather tiresome—children do not like to be uncomfortable every day. Setting a goal gives them a more exact idea of what they are aiming for and when they can stop. It improves motivation.

How to do it: Let's assume your child has been withholding urination for twenty-five to thirty minutes a day. Now, when he first tells you he has to go to the bathroom, set the kitchen timer (or he can set it himself) to his previous record time plus one minute; try to reach the new goal each day. (Indicate new record times on data log.) A small reward may be given for increases in withholding time, e.g., when three or four new records have been reached over a two-week period.

Watch for deconditioning in the child's response to the alarm (see pages 82-83). Sometimes after showing good response to the alarm, a child will no longer respond to it. He doesn't wake up to the alarm—he doesn't hear it. It may be necessary to get a different alarm with a louder or different noise and resume the paired-association exercises (see page 78). You really need to stay on top of this so that the momentum of the conditioned response isn't lost.

What to Expect

At this point, you should see some steady progress: gold stars instead of silver. It is very important to keep encouraging your child not to get overtired, nor to go to bed too late, not to overload with fluids in the evening, and to watch evening snacks. Sometimes there will be a series of dry nights followed by a series of wet nights. (As mentioned above, watch for deconditioning, i.e., your child's no longer hearing the alarm.)

When your child is no longer being awakened after bedtime to go to the bathroom and is earning gold stars 50 percent of the time, move on to Phase IV. See page 93.

Q. My child got up to go to the bathroom, but didn't make it. Does this happen to other children?

A. Many parents have told me about children who get up on their own but do not make it to the bathroom, instead urinating on the floor, in the closet, on the walls—doing some rather strange kinds of things. I actually think this is good news, as strange as it may seem. The poor parents are saying, "Gee whiz, at least before we had the problem, but it was isolated and limited to the bedroom, and now this kid is urinating God only knows where!" What is happening is that the children are responding to signals from bladder contractions or from a full bladder—signals they have never responded to previously. But these kids are only partially awake. They intend to go to the bathroom, but they are out of it, still half asleep. In many instances, we are dealing with a semi-sleepwalking episode: the child may think he is in the bathroom.

The child's intentions are certainly good, and you just need to make sure that you are not in the line of fire. I can assure you that I have never seen this problem persist for any significant length of time. When it happens, it is sometimes difficult to maintain your sense of humor, but that is exactly what I recommend.

Phase IV

In most programs, the criterion for dryness is fourteen consecutive nights of dryness, but I like to see a month. A visual sequencing exercise is introduced at this time as an additional aid in helping your child respond to bladder contractions and in remaining dry. When your child has had two weeks of dryness, begin to wean him from the alarm.

Continue the following:

- Data Log and Dry Nights (Star) Chart (blank forms for Phase IV are provided in the Appendix, pages 106 and 108).

- Midstream-interruption exercise (push-up), *but instead of ten times each urination, do exercise during only one urination each day, preferably in the morning and not at bedtime. Discontinue when child becomes dry.*

- Bladder-stretching structured withholding exercise once daily (see page 91); *discontinue when child is dry for one month.*

- Bladder-capacity measurement twice a week (see pages 54-56); *discontinue when normal capacity is reached or when child becomes dry.*

- Monitoring evening snacks and drinks (see pages 53-54); written record not required. *Continue until child is dry for one month; then, discontinue monitoring gradually. If child wets after drinking carbonated and caffeinated beverages, obviously those should be eliminated from his evening diet.*

- Child's trip to bathroom every night at bedtime, *even after he becomes dry.*

● Nightly alarm use (see pages 77-78 and 79). *See instructions below for weaning child from alarm.*

Introduce visual sequencing technique. This is a mental rehearsal of the night's activities that will help your child to respond to bladder contractions and the feeling of a full bladder—and to remain dry.

How to do it: Every night before bedtime, have your child sit in a comfortable chair. Tell him to take a series of slow, deep breaths and to focus on relaxing and sinking very deeply into the chair. Then, ask him to close his eyes as they start to get heavy. Begin to discuss what will happen during the night. Ask him to concentrate on the feeling of a full bladder, the feeling associated with a need to go to the bathroom. Ask him to imagine that he's asleep and to think what he will do when he feels that happen. Ask him to imagine getting up and going to the bathroom.

Note on data log that exercise has been done. Discontinue visual sequencing when your child becomes dry.

Begin to wean your child from the alarm. *How to do it:* After two weeks of dryness, have your child pick a night of the week that he will sleep without the alarm. (It's best not to pick a weekend night, because children tend to be more tired on the weekends and wetting is more likely to occur.) If your child stays dry without the alarm, he can try sleeping without it two or three nights, then for longer periods. If he wets two nights in a row, go back to using the alarm and repeat the process until your child stays dry for one month.

What to Expect

You still have to be patient. Remember, you are trying to cure a problem that occurred almost every night, probably more than once a night, for years. The average bedwetting case takes approximately three months to reach this level. (If your child was wetting three or four times a night, don't be surprised if it takes six months.)

Visual sequencing: a mental
rehearsal of when to get up
to go to the bathroom.

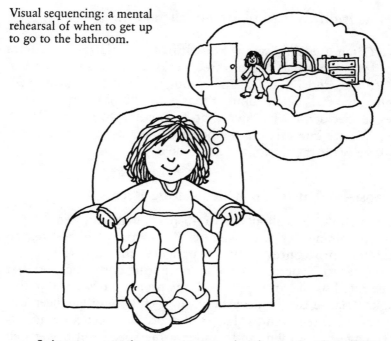

It is very, very important to maintain motivation. Focus on the fact that the severity of the problem is steadily waning and that your child is responding to the treatment. Continue to offer small rewards for progress, and encourage your child to reach his goal of being dry.

When your child has stayed dry for one month, then it's time to celebrate—and time to give him the reward you agreed on at the beginning of the treatment program.

Q. Why is it important to phase out the wetness alarm?

A. The alarm is a noise that the child doesn't like, and there are times when it is like the sword of Damocles hanging over his head—it's the threat of the alarm going off that keeps him dry. We don't want any crutches; we want him to have confidence that even without the alarm he's not going to have an accident. So, we wean him from the wetness alarm.

Q. Is it difficult to phase out the alarm?

A. Often, the child weans himself from the alarm. Sometimes a child who has had two or three weeks of dryness will come in to see me, and I'll say, "You're not wearing the alarm every night, are you?" He'll admit at that point, "No, I'm really not." He has decided on his own that he is going to be dry. That's fine. We are interested in the bottom line, or the bottom sheet, and we want the bottom sheet to be dry.

*   *   *

Relapse—What to Do If Bedwetting Recurs

Studies show that about 20 to 40 percent of children relapse after becoming dry with wetness alarms or other bedwetting treatment procedures. In my experience, the relapse rate has been close to 20 percent in children entering our clinic, and that is the rate I would anticipate with the program described in this book. Relapse can be devastating to a child who has been dry for two or three months. His confidence has been soaring, his self-image has grown, and suddenly the specter of a wet bed rears its ugly head once again.

Relapse is different from an occasional accident, but if wetting occurs on two consecutive nights, *don't wait*: as soon as this happens, go back to instituting midstream-interruption (push-up) and bladder-stretching exercises. If wetting continues, go back to using the alarm. If the child is not responsive to the alarm, go back to awakening him one hour after bedtime to go to the bathroom. Remember the methods that were successful before and use them again.

Sometimes a child will be dry during the winter months and into the spring, and suddenly start wetting again in the summer. Remember the later bedtime that often coincides with Daylight Saving Time, and extra fatigue levels that come with the children's increased activities during the summer months.

Eliminating bedwetting the second time around is usually easier than it was the first time. Compliance is less of a problem because the child remembers that the program worked before, and usually he hates the bedwetting far more than he did the first time.

It is very important to be sensitive to the child and not to let him lose self-esteem. When the problem occurs, tackle it in an unemotional way as a problem-solving experience. Examination of the child by a physician might be useful to ensure that a urinary tract infection is not contributing to the recurrence of the bedwetting, but before taking any major steps to intervene, repeat the treatment program as described above.

4

Treatment for the Older Child and Adult

One to three percent of individuals who are eighteen years old still wet the bed. This means there are quite a few adults who have a problem with bedwetting. In adults, it can cause severe social disruptions and should be treated.

If the bedwetting is primary (it has never really stopped for any extended period of time), then the procedures outlined in this book will be helpful. However, for an adult who wets the bed, it is very important to consider possible medical reasons, such as diabetes, urinary tract infections, and sleep apnea. For that reason, medical evaluation of the bedwetting problem should be sought before starting treatment for the bedwetting itself.

Usually, a young adult or adult doesn't wet the bed three or four times per night as a child might. It is usually once a night and not every night. Sometimes an adult wets only once a week. So, you must ask, "Why doesn't he wet every night?" He clearly has the bladder capacity to be dry, so you might start looking for dietary factors that are contributing to the irritability of the bladder.

If the bedwetting is of a secondary nature, meaning that it has stopped for some time and then started again, this would indicate that some medical or psychological factor is causing it, and professional consultation is indicated.

Stream-interruption and bladder-stretching exercises, as outlined in this book, are quite important in treating the bedwetting problem. For some older individuals, though, there will not be anyone around to help with the PAX (paired association exercise), so they will have to eliminate that. However, since the purpose of the PAX is to teach the individual to respond to the alarm apparatus, and older children and adults generally respond to the alarm and wake up because they don't sleep as deeply as a child, elimination of the exercise isn't a major problem.

With regard to the restriction of caffeinated and carbonated beverages, compliance is often better in the younger child because of the parents' help. But to get an adult to comply with the request to avoid beer or any alcoholic beverage is often quite difficult. It is important to realize that alcohol is a diuretic. It works differently than caffeine, theophylline or theobromine (see discussion on page 68), but it is still a diuretic. Often the adult will avoid alcoholic beverages whenever possible, but they are so often a part of his social environment that sometimes he will continue to drink them in the evening and just pay the price—a wet bed.

Also, often an adult is not sleeping at home and will not wear the alarm regularly. It is important for him to understand the logic behind the use of the alarm—that it is a conditioning device, and in order to be effective, must be used regularly until bedwetting stops.

In quite old people who have lost control of sphincter muscles or of the bladder, stream-interruption exercises are very important in regaining sphincter-muscle control.

Epilogue

Overcoming the bedwetting problem will mean a tremendous boost in your child's self-esteem, and a wonderful feeling of accomplishment for you, the parents, as well as for your child. Curing the bedwetting problem is hard work and demands dedication and persistence. Remember the spontaneous cure rate is only 15 percent a year, so the odds were greatly against you; 85 percent of other children in a similar situation, without treatment, would be expected to still be wetting. Your child and you deserve congratulations for successfully performing this task.

Working with children and their parents in the bedwetting treatment program has been personally rewarding for me. I've had the opportunity to take a negative experience—that is, bedwetting—and turn it into something positive. Often parents seemingly race their children into the office to show me the results of the nightly logs, and sometimes I'm not certain who is prouder, the child or the parent.

The relationship with the children has been especially gratifying. I've learned to assemble and disassemble all of the Transformer toys and I've become quite familiar with the new comic book heroes and heroines.

Most of all the opportunity to help children overcome a problem that causes them to suffer embarrassment and, in some cases, psychological blame, has provided motivation for me. I wish there had been someone to help me with my bedwetting problem when I was growing up, and I feel quite certain that you will appreciate what an important contribution you have made to your child's well being.

Appendix

SUPPLIERS OF WETNESS ALARMS

Alarms may be ordered from the following suppliers and also are available at some retail stores such as drugstores, pharmacies, and home health care or medical supply stores. Prices range from $45 to $70.

Nite Train-r Enterprises Inc., P.O. Box 282, Newberg, OR 97132. 1-800-544-4240 or (503)538-8717. *Nite Train'r II:* alarm box attached to Velcro patch pins to pajama collar or shoulder of tee shirt; moisture-sensing pad worn in underpants. *Ultralert:* same type as Nite Train'r II with louder alarm. Boy's and girl's models.

Nytone Medical Prod. Inc., 2424 S. 900 West, Salt Lake City, UT 84119. (801)973-4090. *Nytone:* alarm fastened to wrist; moisture-sensitive clips fastened to outside of underpants.

Palco, 1595 Soquel Dr., Santa Cruz, CA 95065. (408)476-3151. *Wet-Stop:* buzzer attached to Velcro shoulder patch affixed to shoulder of pajama top; moisture-sensing strip attached to outside of underpants.

J. C. Penney Co. Inc., catalog. *Wet Alarm:* moisture-sensing pad placed beneath bed sheet.

Sears, Roebuck and Co., catalog. *Lite-Alert® Alarm* and *Wee-Alert Alarm:* Both models: alarm box placed on table; moisture-sensing pad placed beneath sheet.

Travis Company, Inc., P.O. Box 5646, 8017 Albacore Ave., Charleston,

OR 97420. 1-800-4 dry bed (national), 1-800-2 dry bed (Oregon) or (503)888-3242. *Wet • No • More*™: alarm in foam material belt worn around waist; urine-sensitive pad worn inside underpants. Female and male models.

CANADIAN SUPPLIERS OF WETNESS ALARMS

Nite Train-r
B C Medical Equipment Ltd.
2106 Main St.
Vancouver, BC V5T 3C5
Canada
(604)876-4186

H & H Care Limited
3429 12th St. NE
Calgary Alta T2E 6S6
Canada
(403)250-2200
Health First Medical Supplies
Ste #101 7080 River Rd.
Richmond BC V6X 1X5
Canada
(604)273-3221

J. Stevens Homecare Products, Ltd.
134 Lakeshore Rd., W.
Oakville, Ontario
L6K 1E4
(416)845-5093

Regency Medical Supply Ltd.
4437 Canada Way
Burnaby, BC V5G 1J3
Canada

Nytone Medical Prod.
Major Medical Supply
685 Main Street E.
Hamilton, Ontario
L8M 1K4
(416)547-0188
Ron Lawrence

Palco
Order directly from Palco in U.S.A.

J.C. Penney
Canadians can order from the U.S. catalog.

Sears, Roebuck & Co.
Sears, Canada, Inc.

Travis Co.
Regent St.-Pierre Inc.
4338 St.-Denis
Montreal, Quebec
H2G 2K8
(514)849-2407

DATA LOG—Phase I

Date	Wet	Dry	Bedtime/ Fell Asleep	Exercises Done: Midstream Interrupt	Bladder Stretch	Bladder Capacity (ounces)	# Daytime Bathroom Trips	Evening Snacks and Drinks

DATA LOG—Phase II

Date	Wet	Dry	Bedtime/Fell Asleep	Wetting Time (alarm sounded) *small wet spot	Exercises Done: Midstream Interrupt/PAX	Bladder Stretch	Bladder Capacity (ounces)	# Daytime Bathroom Trips

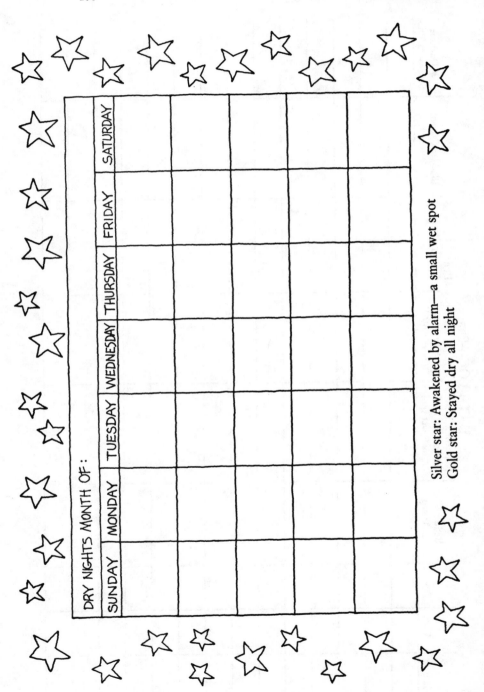

DRY NIGHTS MONTH OF:

SUNDAY	MONDAY	TUESDAY	WEDNESDAY	THURSDAY	FRIDAY	SATURDAY

Silver star: Awakened by alarm—a small wet spot
Gold star: Stayed dry all night

DATA LOG—Phase III

Date	Wet	Dry	Bedtime/ Fell Asleep	Wetting Time (alarm sounded) *small wet spot	Exercises Done:		Bladder Capacity (ounces)	# Daytime Bathroom Trips
					Midstream Interrupt	Bladder Stretch (minutes held)		

DATA LOG—Phase IV

Date	Wet	Dry	Bedtime/ Fell Asleep	Wetting Time (alarm sounded) *small wet spot	Exercises Done:		Bladder Capacity (ounces)	# Daytime Bathroom Trips
					Midstream Interrupt/Vis. Seq.	Bladder Stretch (minutes held)		

REFERENCES

Azrin, Nathan H., and Besalel, Victoria A. *A Parent's Guide to Bedwetting Control*. New York: Pocket Books, 1981

Ferber, Richard. *Solve Your Child's Sleep Problems*. New York: Simon and Schuster, 1985

McLain, Larry G. 1979. "Childhood Enuresis." In *Current Problems in Pediatrics*, vol. 9 (issue 8), June 1979, pp. 1-36. Chicago: Year Book Medical Publishers, Inc.

Mikkelsen, Edwin J., Rapoport, Judith L. "Enuresis: Psychopathology, Sleep Stage, and Drug Response." In *Urologic Clinics of North America, Symposium on Pediatric Urology*, vol. 7, no. 2., June 1980, pp. 361-77.

Olness, Karen. "The Use of Self-Hypnosis in the Treatment of Childhood Nocturnal Enuresis." *Clinical Pediatrics*, March 1975.

Schmitt, Barton D. "Nocturnal Enuresis: An Update on Treatment." In *Pediatric Clinics of North America, Symposium on Persistent Signs and Symptoms*, vol. 29, no. 1, February 1982, pp. 21-36.

Index

About the Author

Martin B. Scharf, Ph.D., received his bachelor's degree from the University of California at Los Angeles and his doctorate in pharmacology from Pennsylvania State University. He has served as associate director of the Sleep Research and Treatment Center and as an assistant professor in the department of psychiatry at the Milton S. Hershey Medical Center at Pennsylvania State University; as director of the Sleep/Wake Disorders Center and assistant professor of psychiatry at the University of Cincinnati Medical Center; and as former associate director of the nation's first sleep clinic at U.C.L.A. He is currently director of the Sleep Disorders Laboratory of The Mercy Hospital in Cincinnati, Ohio, and clinical director of the Sleep/Wake Disorders Unit of The Miami-Valley Hospital in Dayton, Ohio.

Dr. Scharf has published numerous scientific articles about sleep disorders in such prestigious medical journals as *The New England Journal of Medicine* and *The Journal of the American Medical Association*. He is a member of the Sleep Research Society, the Association of Sleep Disorders Centers, the American Federation for Clinical Research, and the American Society of Pharmacologists and Experimental Therapeutics. He is board-certified as a clinical polysomnographer by the Association of Sleep Disorders Centers.

Dr. Scharf has been featured on such national television and radio shows as "20/20" and "Hour Magazine," and in the national newspaper *USA Today*. He lives in Cincinnati with his wife, Lauren, and their two daughters, Rosalyn and Cyvia.

Other Books of Interest
from Writer's Digest Books